Liver Cancer - Multidisciplinary Approach

Edited by Georgios Tsoulfas

Published in London, United Kingdom

Liver Cancer - Multidisciplinary Approach
http://dx.doi.org/10.5772/intechopen.1000387
Edited by Georgios Tsoulfas

Contributors
Anna Garmpi, Christian N. Schill, Christos Damaskos, Daniel Tugume, David Apuulison, Dimitrios Dimitroulis, Ioannis Hatzaras, Ioannis Margaris, James V. Guarrera, Keri E. Lunsford, Lisa O'Kane, Maryam Shafaati, Maryam Zare, Mohammadreza Salehi, Nguyen Hai Nam, Nikolaos Arkadopoulos, Nikolaos Garmpis, Pauline Irumba, Umut Tüysüz, William H. Smith

First published in London, United Kingdom, 2024 by IntechOpen
IntechOpen is the global imprint of INTECHOPEN LIMITED, registered in England and Wales, registration number: 11086078, 167-169 Great Portland Street, London, W1W 5PF, United Kingdom

British Library Cataloguing-in-Publication Data
A catalogue record for this book is available from the British Library

Additional hard and PDF copies can be obtained from orders@intechopen.com

Liver Cancer - Multidisciplinary Approach
Edited by Georgios Tsoulfas
p. cm.
Print ISBN 978-0-85466-995-0
Online ISBN 978-0-85466-994-3
eBook (PDF) ISBN 978-0-85466-996-7

For EU product safety concerns:
IN TECH d.o.o., Prolaz Marije Krucifikse Kozulić 3, 51000 Rijeka, Croatia,
info@intechopen.com or visit our website at intechopen.com.

Meet the editor

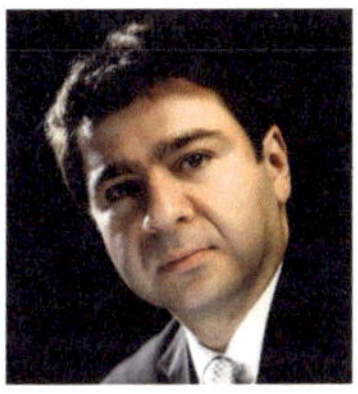

Dr. Georgios Tsoulfas received his MD from Brown University School of Medicine, USA, and completed a general surgery residency at the University of Iowa Hospitals and Clinics, as well as a transplant research fellowship at the Starzl Transplant Institute at the University of Pittsburgh. He then completed a two-year transplantation surgery fellowship at the Massachusetts General Hospital, Harvard Medical School and then joined the Division of Solid Organ Transplantation and Hepatobiliary Surgery at the University of Rochester Medical Center as Associate Professor of Surgery. He has currently moved back to Greece, where he is Professor of Transplantation Surgery and Chief at the Department of Transplantation Surgery, the Aristotle University of Thessaloniki School of Medicine and the Center for Research and Innovation in Solid Organ Transplantation. He has published more than 200 papers in peer-reviewed journals as well as 35 book chapters. He has edited 6 books and is a reviewer for 30 international journals and an editorial board member of several others, including International Surgery and Annals of Surgical Oncology. The recipient of awards such as the Edward E. Mason Award for excellence in patient care and education, Dr. Tsoulfas is a member of several professional organizations including The Transplantation Society (TTS), the American Society of Transplant Surgeons (ASTS), Association for Academic Surgery, International College of Surgeons, American College of Surgeons, International Liver Transplantation Society, Society for Laparoscopic Surgeons, and International HepaticoPancreaticoBilliary Association (IPHBA). He is also the recipient of the American College of Surgeons International Guest Scholarship. He has served as a member of multiple committees, including the International Relations Committee of the American College of Surgeons and the International Relations Committee of the American HepaticoPancreaticoBiliary Association (AHPBA). Dr. Tsoulfas is the president of the Greek Chapter of the International College of Surgeons. Previously, he was World President of the International College of Surgeons and Chair of the International Relations Committee of the American College of Surgeons. He has served as a member of the AHPBA and the IHPBA Education and Training Committees and the E-AHPBA Education Committee (Training Program Accreditation), the ASTS CME committee, and the American Association for the Study of Liver Diseases (AASLD) Training and Workforce Committee. He is also a member of the Executive Council of the Hellenic Surgical Society and President of the Hellenic Transplantation Society. Dr. Tsoulfas' clinical and research interests include hepatobiliary surgery, primary and secondary hepatic malignancies, ischemia/reperfusion injury, solid organ transplantation, as well as medical/surgical education and the use of technology, including applications of artificial technology and 3D printing in surgery.

Contents

Preface

The combination of the globally high prevalence of hepatocellular carcinoma (HCC), the complex nature of hepatic anatomy and physiology, and the continuously increasing wealth of information and techniques regarding its management make HCC one of the most interesting and challenging areas in surgery. As such, it is also an area where a multidisciplinary approach is a necessity, especially given the combined medical and surgical issues that these patients face. The role of the surgeon is critical in the sense that decisions have to be made regarding the different strategies and techniques and which one is best for the specific patient at the specific stage of the disease; however, a multitude of other specialists such as the hepatologist, the radiologist, the interventional radiologist, the oncologist, the intensivist, and the internist, to name a few, play critical roles in planning the care of these patients, whether it has to do with prevention, diagnosis, or management. Additionally, the technological progress that we are witnessing has added several weapons to the armamentarium of the medical and surgical team.

This book provides an overview of the main challenges and opportunities involved in the multidisciplinary management of HCC, whether they have to do with epidemiology, molecular diagnosis, staging, the role of immunotherapy, or, of course, the great variety of surgical techniques and technologies involved in the therapy. Its value lies in the fact that the authors present us with their distilled wisdom, which is the result of substantial experience and daily involvement in this most difficult field of medicine and surgery.

Overall, this book is a useful resource for any physician, whether they are in training or in practice, treating patients with hepatic diseases.

Georgios Tsoulfas, MD, PhD, FICS, FACS
Professor of Transplantation Surgery,
Chief of Department of Transplantation Surgery,
Center for Innovation and Research in Solid Organ Transplantation,
Aristotle University School of Medicine,
Thessaloniki, Greece

Section 1

Advances in Multidisciplinary Approach

Chapter 1

Advances in Multidisciplinary Approach for Liver Cancer

Pauline Irumba, Daniel Tugume and David Apuulison

Abstract

The collective effort of specialized individuals in every institution helps in contributing to the ultimate success. Malignant liver cells mimic similar actions of coordinated efforts through their unregulated multiplication subsequently resulting in multiorgan failure whence the third most common cause of cancer related mortality globally. Irrespective of the form of liver cancer in the patient, there are significant challenges to the patient, carers, and health professionals. Issues arise in line of decision making and implementation of the best management modality. Due to the complexity, and patient's needs during metastatic processes, multidisciplinary input is a necessity for optimal outcomes. Complications arising from liver cancer tend to impair the patient's functioning. To avert poor hastened outcomes for better prognosis, unique interventions should be from specialized professionals. Patients who are treated successfully may require rehabilitation therapy. In instances when liver cancer is incurable, the best quality of life should be maintained while on supportive chemotherapy with integration of palliative care.

Keywords: multidisciplinary, team, liver cancer, health, teamwork, patients

1. Introduction

Liver cancer is one of the most common malignancies contributing to significant morbidity and mortality globally [1]. Histologically, it mainly exists in the forms of hepatocellular carcinoma (HCC) and intrahepatic cholangiocarcinoma (iCCA) although other forms of primary and secondary liver malignancies exist. Globally, HCC remains the most frequent histologic type of primary liver cancer [2, 3]. Development of each of the subtypes is linked to distinct risk factors. Hepatitis B Virus (HBV) and Hepatitis C virus (HCV) have been identified as key risk factors for development of HCC while parasites (*Opisthorchis viverrini* and *Clonorchis sinensis*) have been implicated for iCCA. However alcohol and non-alcoholic steatohepatitis could also increase the risk for liver cancer [4]. Despite the decrease in viral infections overtime, HCC due to non-alcoholic steatohepatitis is gradually increasing. Pathologically, liver cirrhosis has been a key step for liver carcinogenesis in most forms of HCC and iCCA. Cases have been documented across the globe mainly from Africa, Asia, and the Americas, among less developed and developed countries [1, 5]. Cases increase every year with males being more affected than females. The occurrence of liver cancer differs regionally often due to common predisposition; for example liver cirrhosis due to viruses (HBV and HCV) and excessive alcohol consumption was more in parts of Asia, Africa, and Europe, respectively [6].

Due to its aggressiveness, liver cancer remains complicated to treat and manage. This complexity mostly results in poor prognosis especially the overall recuperation following late diagnosis. Mortality due to liver cancer still remains significant even in developed nations with advanced medical care [7, 8]. Individual variations also exist in regard to metastatic process in patients. Estimates indicate that by 2030, almost all countries will have an increased number of individuals with liver cancer except Japan. This calls for a well-trained team of health professionals at all levels to optimize treatment and care [9].

Although there is improvement in the management of cancerous conditions globally, liver cancer in its different forms still remains a challenge. The possible reduction of HCC cases in resource-rich regions was achieved mainly through therapies like resection, ablation, and transplant in the early stages of liver cancer [10, 11]. Recent innovations in therapies for liver cancer including molecular targeted systemic therapies and immunotherapy are being used for intermediate and advanced stages of liver cancer. These interventions improve prognosis if integrated with multidisciplinary efforts [12]. Curative therapies in isolation do not offer the desired cure in all that affected; for example only below 13% can be cured by tumor ablation, surgical resection, and liver transplant [13]. Incorporating different dimensions of care for the patient with liver cancer becomes a vital necessity. Patient care and needs should be through a form of either a lens or prism with the patient at the center. These needs could be internalized or externalized. Interestingly, these needs and care concepts cannot be in a form of one bundle that fits all but rather individualized. Derangements in the different human domains could incidentally destabilize the recuperation process. These human domains could be physiological, psychological, social and spiritual. An imbalance in any human domain affects the overall wellbeing of the patient [14]. Borrowing from the concept of health which is not mere absence of infirmity but rather totality in overall wellbeing, care should seek to address all health problems affecting the patient. Approaches to offer such care to patients with liver cancer while considering their needs should be multidimensional with a specialized team.

2. Multidisciplinary team approach

So, which approach is multidisciplinary? Does it mean interdisciplinary? Does it mean interprofessional? What is transdisciplinary?

Multidisciplinary approach derives from multidisciplinary teamwork. Although the terms multidisciplinary, interdisciplinary, and interprofessional appear similar, they have slight differences. They are often used interchangeably. Several authors have defined multidisciplinary teamwork. It has been described as a mechanism to ensure holistic patient care and service to patients throughout their disease trajectory across all levels of care [15, 16]. Relatedly, multidisciplinary team in oncology has been defined as "a cooperation between different specialized professionals involved in cancer care with the overarching goal of improving treatment efficiency and patient care". Generally a multidisciplinary team entails collective specialized efforts and services toward a patient by members with different training to cater to the patient's diverse needs with the aim of better patient outcomes. With multidisciplinary approach, a patient is assessed and managed individually by several professionals while maintaining their disciplinary boundaries according to the scope of practice. The role(s) of each professional may be either related or unrelated. The relationship between the multidisciplinary team and multidisciplinary approach is similar to that of the chain and the sprocket. A multidisciplinary team approach offers alternatives to team members to implement their roles in order to improve the quality of life of a patient with liver cancer. On the other hand, interdisciplinary approach was defined by [17] as willingness to share specialist knowledge and authority if the needs of the client can be met by other professional groups. There is emphasis on exchange between professional groups. Thus, interdisciplinary is often used interchangeably with interprofessional. During interdisciplinary team working, members share their individual assessments and develop a joint management plan. Transdisciplinary approach entails members of the team sharing roles to achieve common goals. Specialists could share their skills with other members of different specializations in the team. Being almost similar to delegation of tasks in health practice, it could result in task shifting; however, it enables the patient receive the required care in absence required specialist in the team. However, the skills being shared must be appropriate based on the level training and complexity of the of the skill. With this approach, there an individual in the team who should be accountable for the procedures and skills performed on the patient.

3. The team

A therapeutic collaboration among health professionals improves the overall delivery of patient-centered care and subsequent outcomes. Treatment and care are based on the level of the health facility and specialization among the health professionals [18]. Multidisciplinary teams refer to either a group or groups of health professionals from diverse disciplines who come together to provide comprehensive assessment and management for mutual benefit to the patient. The main link in this concept of management is provision of appropriate health services. The team members do not necessarily have to belong to one unit. There should be self-driven specialized input in-line with the patient condition to summate efforts for holistic management of patient. Although the patient has a confirmed diagnosis of liver cancer, different dimensions of both physical and psychological life are affected. This presents with complexity requiring multidisciplinary teamwork; for example, metastasis to distant organs in the body could require specialists of organs affected in the body together with spiritual, financial, and societal dimensions [19, 20].

Multidisciplinary system is comprised of intertwined single or several appointment(s) with a patient scheduled so that several health professionals of different training and skills are involved in each visit. Team members have different roles and specializations. They include nurses, medical doctors, psychologists, social workers, spiritual leaders, investigation experts, and trusted caregiver(s). Team members (**Figure 1**) may vary based on the needs of the patient and staging of liver cancer. Investigation experts may include laboratory team members and radio-imaging experts. In this regard, spirituality and religion should be viewed as distinct concepts. However, one helps achieve the other. It is important to note that an individual may not have a religion but attain spirituality. Religion could help one achieve spirituality. The healthcare professional does not need to impose own beliefs and perceptions on a patient in crisis due to liver cancer [21].

Training about multidisciplinary approach of management is important in order to achieve optimal results. This could be curriculum based and in service training. Interprofessional education seeks to educate health professionals within their core specialization about all important aspects of the patient's life. It helps health

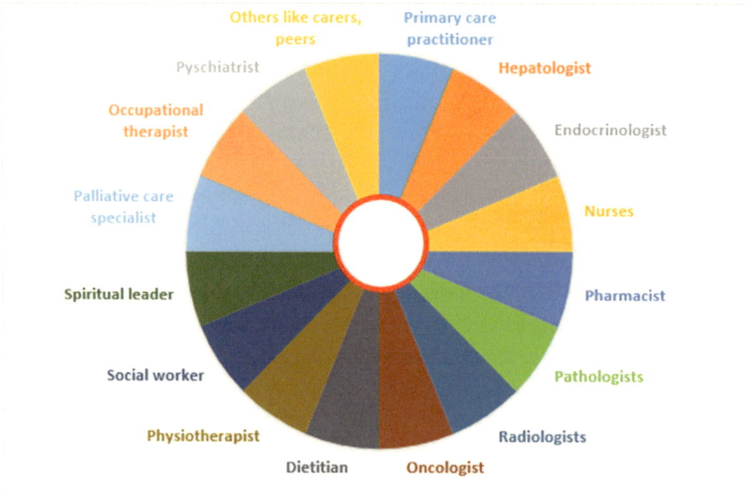

Figure 1.
Multidisciplinary health professional team members "The Multidisciplinary Wheel".

professionals realize the uniqueness of every patient encountered [22]. Liver cancer affects different aspects of life, which requires distinct specialized knowledge for management. In this training, every member learns to appreciate the need of other members who are empowered with decision making on the patient care plan. Inefficiency in management of liver cancer patients may arise not only from individual deficiency of knowledge and skills but also from inefficiency in the team [23]. A training program that utilizes case-based scenarios, simulations, critical thinking, analysis, communication skills, description of roles, and support should be established in health institutions caring for liver cancer patients. These programs should have a feasible framework that suits needs and gaps identified in the setting [24, 25]. This approach has been limited by lack of perceived value, tight schedules, lack of flexibility in the curriculum, poor attitude among health professionals, lack of awareness by key stakeholders, and limited resources for interprofessional training [22]. Efforts should be tailored at implementing and building a multidisciplinary team (**Figure 1**) while identifying barriers to the process and creating feasible solutions to such hurdles.

In this continuum of care, the patient is at the center of care, being the most important person in the team. Like a fulcrum, the progression of events revolves around his/her overall well-being and satisfaction. This requires routine evaluation in the quality of care offered to the patient. A member in the multidisciplinary team preferably the primary care practitioner or advanced nurse should help coordinate this care.

4. Why multidisciplinary team approach?

The main aim of a multidisciplinary team is to provide optimal coordinated patient care and management. As such, the team requires good leadership [26, 27]. Multidisciplinary team approach is effective for individuals with complex care needs and long-term debilitating conditions in liver cancer. Multidisciplinary approach has been associated with improved overall survival of patients with liver cancer. This not

Health profession	Roles
Primary care practitioner	Surveillance of all forms of liver cancer
Hepatologist	Treatment of all of liver-associated disorders, liver transplant
Endocrinologist	Identification of high-risk patients for liver cancer
Nurses	Multifaceted roles to improve care
Pharmacists	Guidance on medications, drug interactions, optimizing treatment
Pathologist	Confirm the diagnosis of liver cancer, staging, and its subtype.
Radiologist	Perform imaging studies, interventional radiology, and radiotherapy when preferred
Oncologist	Specialist in treatment of cancer like surgical oncologist, medical oncologist.
Dietitian	Guide the patient on dietary modification and lifestyle
Physiotherapist	Offer physical therapy to help regain strength, physical function thereby improve the level of independence in activities of daily living.
Occupational therapist	Help patients overcome effects of treatment such as chemotherapy and keep engaged mentally to improve their cognition and functionality.
Social worker	Resource mobilization, explaining diagnosis and management plan, liaising with healthcare team, support caregivers.
Spiritual/religious leader	Provide a calm environment, coping mechanism for positive living while undergoing treatment. Techniques such as meditation, counseling sessions, prayers sessions, encouragement, and mindfulness could be used.
Palliative care specialists	Care to improve quality of life, prolong during terminal stages of liver cancer.
Psychiatrist	Prevention, early detection, and treatment of psychiatric illnesses.
Others like peers, carers	Social support network, help with household activities, help with activities of daily living like washing and bathing, monitor for side effects, assist in administration of medications, organize and keep medical records, schedule appointments.

Table 1.
The multidisciplinary team in the management of a patient with liver cancer.

only improves the quality of life but also lower mortality burden despite requiring more medical resources compared to conventional cancer management.

There are higher chances of receiving appropriate care for patients under multidisciplinary care compared to those under conventional cancer management [28].

During the terminal stages of liver cancer, maintenance of meaningful life is best achieved through basic activities of daily living and physical and cognitive function [29, 30]. This is mostly achievable through multidisciplinary team approach, which still remains a distant dream in several nations globally especially the developing nations. Even in the developed world, minority groups of elderly patients under palliative care face exclusion when it comes to access to multidisciplinary specialists mostly due to being mentally handicapped. **Table 1** includes a summary of distinct roles by multidisciplinary team members.

5. Factors that influence multidisciplinary team working

Multidisciplinary team approach can be challenging for the team members especially if certain parameters are not fullfilled. Several research studies [31] have reported a number of factors influencing team work among team members in health facilities. They were categorized into 7, which included; preparation, health professional attendance, caregiver attendance, schedule, meeting, discipline, administrative support, cases and streamlining. The health institution's input should cultivate a culture to enable a belief about the benefits of multidisciplinary team discussion, technology, required skills, motivation to provide the required quality care, and collegiality among health professionals [32]. Other notable factors include communication techniques, presence of multidisciplinary models, health system with policies that support multidisciplinary team approach, and patient-related information [33, 34].

6. Multidisciplinary approach in the management of cancer

To achieve optimal benefits of multidisciplinary team work, certain models could be used. This enables discussion of complex cases with appropriate actions. The discussion to guide proper decision making and informed management could range from patients with suspected liver cancer, confirmed liver cancer and those on treatment. The model advocated for could be developed either in national or international guidelines. Modification could be done with expert consultation to integrate the local needs and emerging demands of liver cancer patients being cared for. Modification could also consider the resource demands, availability, and limitations. Increased workload due to increasing cases of liver with few health professionals could make efforts of multidisciplinary approach futile [35, 36]. The following models are crucial for multidisciplinary team working for liver cancer patients.

Capability model: This determines whether an individual could accomplish an assigned task in both theory and practice. It explores the competences of an individual to guide. Professions in the team bring together their unique skills. Competencies vary according to their experience and qualifications.

Care management: also referred to as case management. This model aims at helping patients survive and optimize their adjustment to the community. Case management contains distinct models including clinical case management, strengths model, intensive case management model, brokerage model, assertive community treatment model, and rehabilitatation models. Each model contains different specialists with an overall leader and coordinator. Brokerage mainly involves coordinating services often with non-clinically trained individuals. As such, the other models (clinical case management, strength, intensive case, assertive community treatment and rehabilitation) are useful in multidisciplinary team work [37–39].

With recent advances in laparoscopic liver resection, surgical resection remains the mainstay for HCC for several decades. It can be considered for patients with non-metastatic disease and normal underlying liver function. Patients with compensated cirrhosis with no evidence of portal hypertension could also benefit from this therapy. Resection must also be performed in a way that maximizes recovery while minimizing post-operative complications and adverse outcomes [7, 40]. To optimize outcomes, multidisciplinary approach and models should be utilized. The perioperative process should involve members of different specializations and training. This slightly differs from the traditional method of management focused on the surgical, medical, and chemotherapeutic interventions where the ultimate decision rested upon the lead physician. Preparation of the patient in the preoperative phase entails all members of the multidisciplinary team. With a coordinator, regular meetings are organized with the patient and significant others. Thorough explanation ultimately keeps both the patient and carers in the know. An informed patient is an expert patient who can cooperate and work toward own better life. Roles of the patient under multidisciplinary care aim at respect, shared decision making and patient empowerment. Efforts should focus on building their understanding while integrating their expectations [41, 42]. Team work must be carried out throughout phases of perioperative care (preoperative, intraoperative, and post-operative). A number of liver resection procedures can be employed in management of liver cancer with promising results. These procedures include non-anatomical resection, segmentectomy, bi-segmentectomy, major resection, and extended major resection. However, some rules must be respected: the future liver remnant (FLR) must have an adequate afferent and efferent blood supply, and biliary drainage. Furthermore, the volume of FLR must be sufficient to maintain a liver function during the postoperative period [43].

Adjuvant therapy after HCC resection in early stages holds promising potential as it may eradicate residual cancer cells and prevent secondary liver carcinogenesis. Several adjuvant strategies have been tested in clinical trials, including systemic and intra-arterial chemotherapy, intra-arterial radiolabeled lipiodol, TACE (trans-arterial chemoembolization), acyclic retinoids, interferon, adoptive immunotherapy, autologous tumor vaccine, and, more recently, sorafenib [7]. Postoperative adjuvant chemotherapy helps reduce or eliminate cancerous cells whence increase chances of survival. Use of adjuvant chemotherapy may be limited in some patients with adverse events like adverse reactions to sorafenib. Management of these adverse reactions requires expert consultation including physicians and pharmacists often necessitating permanent discontinuation [44, 45]. Risks and benefits should be weighed while using adjuvant chemotherapy. Decision from this analytical approach should emerge from a technical informed point of view preferably with use of models (**Figure 2**). Adjuvant chemotherapy should not be an option if the risks for its use in the patient outweigh the benefits. Evaluating the risks and benefits of each adjuvant therapeutic agent could help ascertain the overall prognosis. With higher overall survival, the patient could be maintained on appropriate therapy [46, 47]. Medications should be titrated to obtain the maximum therapeutic dose while minimizing its toxicity. Patients should be routinely monitored for both side effects and adverse events. Health professionals should be trained to monitor and identify significant pathophysiological deviations

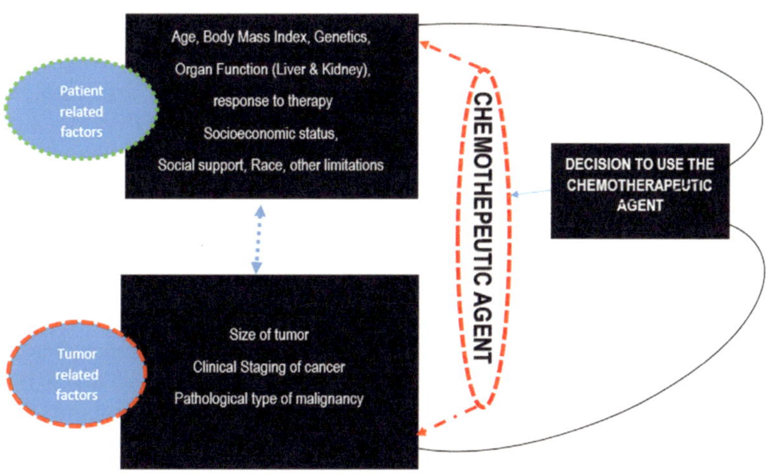

Figure 2.
Risk-benefit model for use of post-operative chemotherapeutic agents.

due to therapy. Liver transplantation (LT), which is usually indicated for patients with poor liver function, has also become safer following advances in perioperative management. Currently, efforts are being made to further expand the indications for liver transplant. Tumor characteristics, including serum alpha-fetoprotein, the presence of microvascular invasion, tumor grade or differentiation, and largest tumor size, are among the most important predictors of recurrence after liver transplant. Bridging therapy to downstage the tumor before LT is also proposed with atezolizumab plus bevacizumab resulting in a better progression-free survival than sorafenib [48].

Computer-based technologies through models of electronic Health (eHealth), for example telemedicine, telenursing, and patient reminder applications, can be a focal point for integrating treatment and care for patients with liver cancer [49]. Several interventions to optimize patient health have been achieved through messaging applications between patients and the healthcare providers. It is much easier to share electronic data about the patient for expert consultation among team members. Websites with key liver cancer patient information for example lifestyle, dietary restrictions and booking appointments can play a crucial role in improving the quality of care, and life among patients with liver cancer [49–52]. Models using telehealth for post-operative patients following liver transplant have been recommended for their ability to improve clinical outcomes [53–55]. Telehealth is also vital in areas with poor access to liver cancer specialty. Telehealth platforms often enable patients open up to express their needs while on therapy in and out of the treatment center. The multidisciplinary team members could also monitor the patient's clinical and psychological status by sharing signs and symptoms from the patient to healthcare providers [56–58].

Risk-benefits models may be adjusted to suit the best patient's needs at the point of diagnosis, and thereafter in the course of management. Chemotherapeutic agents may not be used if they worsen the clinical status of the patient and hasten poor prognosis. A conflict may exist on important needs coexisting at the same time. Those are the scenarios when judgment is guided through expert opinion from members of the multidisciplinary team. The Maslow's hierarchy of needs could be considered to guide their decision.

7. Ethical considerations

Confirmation of liver cancer affects the psychological status of every patient diagnosed. This results in denial that can affect decisions that will be considered thereafter. Therapeutic modalities like chemotherapy and surgery are often viewed as an added burden by patients. Therefore from the patient's perspective, explanations about procedure by the interventionist (surgeon, radiologist, oncologist) are often not understood. Clarity that could be added by other multidisciplinary team members such as the nurses and social workers improves the overall acceptance of therapy [59]. Multidisciplinary team working is a partnership with the goal of improving the patient outcomes when faced with liver cancer. The collaboration among professionals is mainly on mutual agreements and rarely involves legal binding except adhering to the scope of practice. A legal framework solely for guiding multidisciplinary teamwork still lacks in many health institutions. Even when they exist, they are in few health institutions in developed countries [60]. Multidisciplinary team members are often not aware of their medico-legal obligations. This puts several professionals involved in care of liver cancer patients in uncertainity especially those newly integrated in this form of patient care [61]. Key ethical issues identified in multidisciplinary team meetings include duty of care, privacy during meetings, consent of patients, expression of conflicting views, and professional liability. In practice policies should be formulated to guide on the common ethical issues in multidisciplinary team working [61–63].

8. Conflict management during multidisciplinary teamwork

Despite the importance of multidisciplinary teamwork in the management of liver cancer, it often result in conflicts among team members resulting in stress. Ultimately a stressed and strained workforce affects the quality of care offered to patients with liver cancer [64–67], like the saying "When the elephants fight, the grass suffers the consequences". Although the conflicts may not involve actual fights, disagreements in the management plan alone do not benefit the patient. A pre-existing plan for identification of conflicts and their subsequent management should be provided for guidance. Interventions including training on leadership, teamwork, team building, and role training have been used as strategies to prevent conflicts in hospitals and specialized healthcare settings [68, 69]. Whenever faced with conflicts among multidisciplinary team members, evidence based interventions should be used to resolve disputes. Measures to de-escalate tensions, include use of the concept of mindfulness, emotional intelligence, workplace reporting system, effective communication with mediation from friends, and stress management [70, 71].

9. Conclusion

Multidisciplinary team work is necessary for better management of patients with liver cancer. It is crucial to integrate a multidimensional form of care where both physician and non-physician professionals' expertise is considered vital with a patient being the centre of focus. Team members need to acknowledge and appreciate distinct roles of each member and how it contributes significantly to improved quality of life of the patient. Regular trainings ultimately improve the functionality of the multidisciplinary team while reducing chances of conflicts, and poor patient care. Modification of multidisciplinary approach models and techniques to fit the needs of a setup should be routinely done for optimal clinical outcomes of patients with liver cancer.

Acknowledgements

We acknowledge Mountains of the Moon University for providing a conducive environment to prepare this chapter.

Conflict of interest

All authors declare no conflict of interest.

Author details

Pauline Irumba*, Daniel Tugume and David Apuulison
Mountains of the Moon University, Fort Portal, Uganda

*Address all correspondence to: rumbahot.93@gmail.com

References

[1] Rumgay H et al. Global, regional and national burden of primary liver cancer by subtype. European Journal of Cancer. 2022;**161**:108-118

[2] Sohn W et al. Obesity and the risk of primary liver cancer: A systematic review and meta-analysis. Clinical and Molecular Hepatology. 2021;**27**(1):157

[3] Turati F et al. Alcohol and liver cancer: A systematic review and meta-analysis of prospective studies. Annals of Oncology. 2014;**25**(8):1526-1535

[4] Huang DQ et al. Changing global epidemiology of liver cancer from 2010 to 2019: NASH is the fastest growing cause of liver cancer. Cell Metabolism. 2022;**34**(7):969-977 e2

[5] Shi JF et al. Is it possible to halve the incidence of liver cancer in China by 2050? International Journal of Cancer. 2021;**148**(5):1051-1065

[6] Alberts CJ et al. Worldwide prevalence of hepatitis B virus and hepatitis C virus among patients with cirrhosis at country, region, and global levels: A systematic review. The Lancet Gastroenterology & Hepatology. 2022;**7**(8):724-735

[7] Liu C-Y, Chen K-F, Chen P-J. Treatment of liver cancer. Cold Spring Harbor Perspectives in Medicine. 2015;**5**(9):a021535

[8] Gravitz L. Liver cancer. Nature. 2014;**516**(7529):S1-S1

[9] Valery PC et al. Projections of primary liver cancer to 2030 in 30 countries worldwide. Hepatology. 2018;**67**(2):600-611

[10] Colombo M, Maisonneuve P. Controlling liver cancer mortality on a global scale: Still a long way to go. Journal of Hepatology. 2017;**67**(2):216-217

[11] Liver EAFTSOT. EASL–EORTC clinical practice guidelines: Management of hepatocellular carcinoma. Journal of Hepatology. 2012;**56**(4):908-943

[12] Samant H, Amiri HS, Zibari GB. Addressing the worldwide hepatocellular carcinoma: Epidemiology, prevention and management. Journal of Gastrointestinal Oncology. 2021;**12**(Suppl. 2):S361

[13] Mak L-Y et al. Global epidemiology, prevention, and management of hepatocellular carcinoma. American Society of Clinical Oncology Educational Book. 2018;**38**:262-279

[14] Maslow AH. A Theory of Human Motivation.pdf. 1943

[15] Jefferies H, Chan K. Multidisciplinary team working: Is it both holistic and effective? International Journal of Gynecologic Cancer. 2004;**14**:210-211

[16] Taberna M et al. The multidisciplinary team (MDT) approach and quality of care. Frontiers in Oncology. 2020;**10**:85

[17] Carrier J, Kendall I. Professionalism and interprofessionalism in health and community care: Some theoretical issues. In: Owens P, Carrier J, Horder J, editors. Interprofessional Issues in Community and Primary Health Care. 1st ed. London: Palgrave; 1995. DOI: 10.1007/978-1-349-13236-2_2

[18] McLaney E et al. A framework for interprofessional team collaboration in a hospital setting: Advancing team competencies and behaviours. In: Healthcare Management Forum. Los Angeles, CA: SAGE Publications; 2022

[19] Wan CS, Mitchell J, Maier AB. A multidisciplinary, community-based program to reduce unplanned hospital admissions. Journal of the American Medical Directors Association. 2021;**22**(6):1331. e1-1331. e9

[20] Penner J et al. 6-month multidisciplinary follow-up and outcomes of patients with paediatric inflammatory multisystem syndrome (PIMS-TS) at a UK tertiary paediatric hospital: A retrospective cohort study. The Lancet Child & Adolescent Health. 2021;**5**(7):473-482

[21] Ferrell BR, NC, Paice J. Oxford Textbook of Palliative Care Nursing. USA: Oxford University Press; 2015

[22] Shamsher S et al. Multidisciplinary team approach in patient management mandates inclusion of interprofessional education in curriculum. SBV Journal of Basic, Clinical and Applied Health Science. 2021;**4**(4):87-89

[23] Deering S, Johnston LC, Colacchio K. Multidisciplinary teamwork and communication training. Seminars in Perinatology (Elsevier). 2011;**35**(2):89-96. DOI: 10.1053/j.semperi.2011.01.009

[24] Hulse AL. A multidisciplinary learning approach: Training, preparation and role transition. British Journal of Nursing. 2022;**31**(8):430-440

[25] Sowole L et al. High Consequence Infectious Diseases (HCID): The conception and development of a multidisciplinary, interprofessional simulation training programme. Journal of Hospital Infection. 2024;**147**:87-97

[26] Gola M et al. Educational challenges in healthcare design: Training multidisciplinary professionals for future hospitals and healthcare. Annali di Igiene Medicina Preventiva e di Comunità. 2020;**32**(5):549-566

[27] Wang HH. Taking a multidisciplinary team approach to better healthcare outcomes for society. Hong Kong Medical Journal. 2020;**26**(6):551-552

[28] Oh JH, Sinn DH. Multidisciplinary approach for hepatocellular carcinoma patients: Current evidence and future perspectives. Journal of Liver Cancer. 2024;**24**(1):47

[29] Scialla S et al. Rehabilitation for elderly patients with cancer asthenia: Making a transition to palliative care. Palliative Medicine. 2000;**14**(2):121-127

[30] Sekine R et al. Changes in and associations among functional status and perceived quality of life of patients with metastatic/locally advanced cancer receiving rehabilitation for general disability. American Journal of Hospice and Palliative Medicine. 2015;**32**(7):695-702

[31] Walraven JE et al. Factors influencing the quality and functioning of oncological multidisciplinary team meetings: Results of a systematic review. BMC Health Services Research. 2022;**22**(1):829

[32] Maharaj AD et al. Barriers and enablers to the implementation of multidisciplinary team meetings: A qualitative study using the theoretical domains framework. BMJ Quality & Safety. 2021;**30**(10):792-803

[33] Wang C et al. Factors influencing clinical pharmacists' integration into the clinical multidisciplinary care team. Frontiers in Pharmacology. 2023;**14**:1202433

[34] Rosell L, Wihl J, Nilbert M, Malmström M. Health professionals' views on key enabling factors and barriers of national multidisciplinary team meetings in cancer care: A qualitative

study. Journal of Multidisciplinary Healthcare. 2020;**13**:179-186. DOI: 10.2147/JMDH.S240140

[35] Winters DA et al. The cancer multidisciplinary team meeting: In need of change? History, challenges and future perspectives. BJU International. 2021;**128**(3):271-279

[36] Vetere A. Bio/Psycho/Social Models and Multidisciplinary Team Working-Can Systemic Thinking Help? Thousand Oaks, CA: Sage Publications; 2007. pp. 5-12

[37] a Bháird CN et al. Multidisciplinary team meetings in community mental health: A systematic review of their functions. Mental Health Review Journal. 2016;**21**(2):119-140

[38] Söylemez M, Tarhan A. The use of maturity/capability frameworks for healthcare process assessment and improvement. In: Clarke P, O'Connor R, Rout T, Dorling A, editors. Software Process Improvement and Capability Determination. SPICE 2016. Communications in Computer and Information Science. Vol. 609. Cham: Springer; 2016. DOI: 10.1007/978-3-319-38980-6_3

[39] Saint-Pierre C, Herskovic V, Sepúlveda M. Multidisciplinary collaboration in primary care: a systematic review. Family Practice. 2018;**35**(2):132-141

[40] Orcutt ST, Anaya DA. Liver resection and surgical strategies for management of primary liver cancer. Cancer Control. 2018;**25**(1):1073274817744621

[41] Sacristán JA, Aguarón A, Avendaño-Solá C, Garrido P, Carrión J, Gutiérrez A, et al. Patient involvement in clinical research: Why, when, and how. Patient Preference and Adherence. 2016;**10**:631-640. DOI: 10.2147/PPA.S104259

[42] Holm A, Rodkjær LØ, Bekker HL. Integrating patient involvement interventions within clinical practice: A mixed-methods study of health care professional reasoning. MDM Policy & Practice. 2024;**9**(1):23814683241229987

[43] Rabinel P et al. Management of liver cancer. The surgeon's point of view. Reports of Practical Oncology and Radiotherapy. 2017;**22**(2):176-180

[44] Welker M et al. Efficacy and safety of sorafenib in advanced hepatocellular carcinoma under daily practice conditions. Journal of Chemotherapy. 2010;**22**(3):205-211

[45] Tovoli F et al. Management of adverse events with tailored sorafenib dosing prolongs survival of hepatocellular carcinoma patients. Journal of Hepatology. 2019;**71**(6):1175-1183

[46] Halabi S, Li C, Luo S. Developing and validating risk assessment models of clinical outcomes in modern oncology. JCO Precision Oncology. 2019;**3**:1-12

[47] Bullock JM, Lin T, Bilic S. Clinical pharmacology tools and evaluations to facilitate comprehensive dose finding in oncology: A continuous risk-benefit approach. The Journal of Clinical Pharmacology. 2017;**57**:S105-S115

[48] Maki H, Hasegawa K. Advances in the surgical treatment of liver cancer. Bioscience Trends. 2022;**16**(3):178-188

[49] WHO. Country Case Studies on Primary Health Care: China: Multidisciplinary Teams and Integrated Service Delivery across Levels of Care. World Health Organization; 2018

[50] Serper M et al. Multidisciplinary teams, efficient communication, procedure services, and telehealth improve cirrhosis care: A qualitative

study. Hepatology Communications. 2023;7(6):e0157

[51] Aghdam MRF, Vodovnik A, Hameed RA. Role of telemedicine in multidisciplinary team meetings. Journal of Pathology Informatics. 2019;**10**(1):35

[52] Heidelbaugh JJ. Telehealth: A Multidisciplinary Approach: Clinics Collections. Elsevier; 2021

[53] Ertel AE, Kaiser T, Shah SA. Using telehealth to enable patient-centered care for liver transplantation. JAMA Surgery. 2015;**150**(7):674-675

[54] John BV et al. Use of telehealth expedites evaluation and listing of patients referred for liver transplantation. Clinical Gastroenterology and Hepatology. 2020;**18**(8):1822-1830. e4

[55] Hui S, Sane N, Wang A, et al. Hepatocellular carcinoma surveillance in the telehealth era: A single-centre review. Journal of Telemedicine and Telecare. 2023. DOI: 10.1177/1357633X231166032

[56] Serper M, Volk ML. Current and future applications of telemedicine to optimize the delivery of care in chronic liver disease. Clinical Gastroenterology and Hepatology. 2018;**16**(2):157-161. e8

[57] Henson JB et al. Access to technology to support telehealth in areas without specialty care for liver disease. Hepatology. 2023;**77**(1):176-185

[58] Muftah et al. Telehealth interventions in patients with chronic liver diseases: A systematic review. Hepatology. July 2023;**78**(1):179-194. DOI: 10.1097/HEP.0000000000000265

[59] Scott B. Multidisciplinary team approach in cancer care: A review of the latest advancements. Oncology. 2021;**9**(9):2-13

[60] Boumil MM, Freitas DF, Frietas CF. Multidisciplinary representation of patients: The potential for ethical issues and professional duty conflicts in the medical-legal partnership model. Journal of Health Care Law & Policy. 2010;**13**:107

[61] Karas PL, Rankin NM, Stone E. Medicolegal considerations in multidisciplinary cancer care. JTO Clinical and Research Reports. 2020;**1**(4):100073

[62] Sidhom M, Poulsen M. Group decisions in oncology: Doctors' perceptions of the legal responsibilities arising from multidisciplinary meetings. Journal of Medical Imaging and Radiation Oncology. 2008;**52**(3):287-292

[63] Evans AC et al. Medicolegal implications of a multidisciplinary approach to cancer care: Consensus recommendations from a national workshop. Medical Journal of Australia. 2008;**188**(7):401-404

[64] Oliver D, Watson S. Multidisciplinary care. End of Life Care in Neurological Disease. 2013;**14**(11):113-132

[65] Başoğul C. Conflict management and teamwork in workplace from the perspective of nurses. Perspectives in Psychiatric Care. 2021;**57**(2):610-619

[66] Belrhiti Z, Van Belle S, Criel B. How medical dominance and interprofessional conflicts undermine patient-centred care in hospitals: Historical analysis and multiple embedded case study in Morocco. BMJ Global Health. 2021;**6**(7):e006140

[67] Mayaki S, Stewart M. Teamwork, professional identities, conflict, and industrial action in Nigerian healthcare. Journal of Multidisciplinary Healthcare. 2020;**13**:1223-1234

[68] White BAA et al. Conflict management education in the intensive

care unit. American Journal of Critical Care. 2020;**29**(6):e135-e138

[69] Assi MD, Eshah NF, Rayan A. The relationship between mindfulness and conflict resolution styles among nurse managers: A cross-sectional study. SAGE Open Nursing. 2022;**8**:23779608221142371

[70] Somani R et al. A systematic review: Effectiveness of interventions to de-escalate workplace violence against nurses in healthcare settings. Safety and Health at Work. 2021;**12**(3):289-295

[71] Kilag OK et al. Administrators' conflict management and strategies. International Multidisciplinary Journal of Research for Innovation, Sustainability, and Excellence (IMJRISE). 2024;**1**(1):60-67

Chapter 2

Revolutionizing HCV Therapy: microRNA Approaches in New Era of Treatment

Maryam Shafaati, Mohammadreza Salehi and Maryam Zare

Abstract

Since the development and evolution of COVID-19 immunization, the use of mRNA-based technologies has led to revolutionary changes due to the potential of RNA-based therapies, which are believed to be useful in treating many infectious diseases. Information on the treatment of hepatitis C virus (HCV) following this rule highlights the potential therapeutic use of microRNAs (miRNAs). The advent of direct-acting antivirals (DAAs) has changed the paradigm of HCV treatment. However, challenges remain, particularly in the areas of viral resistance, genetic diversity, and chronic diseases. Among these, miRNAs are a sensible approach to complementing and improving existing models. The implementation of new non-coding RNAs should be investigated. This chapter discusses the potential and public awareness of non-coding RNA (ncRNA) strategies against HCV. From the modification of miRNAs to the discovery of non-coding RNA pathways and focusing on their applications, efficacy, and therapeutic potential in HCV. As the scientific community looks toward the development of antiviral drugs, this chapter demonstrates that the introduction of non-coding RNA drugs into existing health systems holds promise for addressing and providing solutions to challenges such as drug resistance, viral persistence, and more. New non-coding RNAs in HCV therapy not only expand the scope of treatment but also define the therapeutic landscape and increase flexibility and adaptability in the face of HCV challenges.

Keywords: hepatitis C virus (HCV), mRNA, miRNAs, HCV therapy, DAA, ncRNA

1. Introduction

1.1 The current state of HCV therapy

Hepatitis C virus (HCV) is a liver-affecting viral infection that is highly prevalent and has a significant impact on people's health worldwide. As such, it is considered a major global health concern [1]. In 1989, American researchers made a breakthrough discovery. They were able to identify a new virus. This virus was isolated from the serum of patients with non-A and non-B hepatitis and was officially named hepatitis

C or HCV [2]. Hepatitis C virus is a small, enveloped, positive-sense, single-stranded RNA virus that belongs to the *Flaviviridae* family and genus *Hepacivirus*. The untranslated regions, 3′-UTR and 5′-UTR, found at both ends of the HCV genome are crucial to both replications of the virus. The internal ribosome entry site (IRES), which is a part of the 5′-UTR, is the internal ribosome binding site that creates a polyprotein that has about 3010 amino acids (9.6 kb). This polyprotein is cleaved by cellular and viral proteases into three structural regions (Core, E1, and E2) and seven viral nonstructural proteins, including P7 and NS2, NS3, NS4 A/B, and NS5 A/B [3].

This life-threatening virus can cause a type of acute (short-term) or chronic (long-term) viral hepatitis that can be associated with liver fibrosis and failure and even some cancers such as hepatocellular carcinoma (HCC) and lymphoma [4]. Acute HCV infections are usually asymptomatic and do not cause fatalities. Within 6 months, 15–20% of infected individuals can recover without treatment. The remaining 70% of those affected (55–85%) will become chronically infected with HCV. Within 20 years, there is a 15–30% risk of cirrhosis among people with a persistent HCV infection. Around 58 million people worldwide are infected with the chronic hepatitis C virus, with an annual total of about 1.5 million new infections. Patients with chronic hepatitis C (CHC) are at a high risk of developing liver cirrhosis, progressive fibrosis, and even HCC if they are not treated [5]. Prevention of HCV infection involves reducing bloodstream transmission risk and public health measures to prevent spread in high-risk communities, including injection drug users. The most commonly reported strategy for contracting HCV infections is intravenous drug abuse [6]. Choo and colleagues sequenced HCV's genome, proposing a comprehensive nomenclature system for genotypes and subtypes based on similarity to various genetic groups, known as genotypes (with 60% nucleotide similarity) and their subtypes (76–80% nucleotide similarity) [7]. A set of genetic variants that differ in each patient but have 90–99% nucleotide similarity is referred to as a quasi-species. The genetic composition of quasi-species results from mutations that occur during viral replication. The elimination of one quasi-species leads to the formation of another because the HCV virus might include incorrect or imperfect copies of its sequence during replication and could evade the immune system's response through continuous mutation. For many people, this is one of the reasons for chronic hepatitis C. Quasi-species have a significant impact on the progression of the disease and how it responds to treatment [8].

There are eight primary genotypes and 86 subtypes of HCV. The distributions of HCV genotypes and subtypes differ throughout regions worldwide. Genotypes 1, 2, and 3 are widely distributed throughout the world. Genotypes 4 and 5 are found in East Africa, South Africa, and Arab countries; genotypes 6 through 8 are found in Southeast Asia, the Democratic Republic of the Congo, and Punjab (India). HCV genotypes significantly influence treatment response rates, aiding in drug selection and duration [9].

Before the discovery of HCV, scientists emphasized the effect of IFN-alpha on the treatment of chronic viral liver diseases. Immune cells naturally produce IFN-alpha in response to viral infections or other stressors. This interferon can create an "interference" against the viral replication and finally protects the host cells from spreading the infection [10]. Since 1984, an experimental study of IFN has been started on the treatment of non-A and non-B hepatitis viral hepatitis. Scientists administered daily doses of IFN-alpha to patients for 16 weeks and measured viral status and liver parameters through blood tests. This experiment brought immediate and impressive results. While some patients showed a minimal response to IFN-alpha treatment and others experienced relapse, half of the participants showed a complete response to the trial [11]. The introduction of HCV was accompanied by extensive research focused on determining the molecular structure of the virus, these studies were able to take a fundamental step in designing drugs that can target specific components of the virus and prevent its replication [12]. In additional studies, it was seen that combination therapy containing IFN-alpha and other antiviral drugs such as ribavirin has more promising results [13, 14]. By altering the nucleoside supply (by decreasing NS5B polymerase activity), ribavirin, a guanosine analog and potent inhibitor of cellular inosine dehydrogenase monophosphate, inhibits the viral replication and subsequently maintains the balance between Th1 and Th2 [15]. Another significant advance in the treatment of HCV came when scientists chemically modified IFN-alpha to increase its duration in the body, called "pegylated" IFN. Finally, the combination of "pegylated" IFN with ribavirin became the standard of care for patients with hepatitis C [16]. The combination of PEG-IFN allows the drug to create a suitable therapeutic interval between interferon injection and facilitating treatment. Combining PEG-INF and ribavirin resulted in sustained viral response levels or SVR (SVR means 100-fold reduction of the viral replication or permanent elimination of the virus) of approximately 42–46% of patients with genotypes 1 and 4 of the virus, and 76–82% for those with genotypes 2 and 3 [17]. Antiviral treatment for HCV genotypes lasts 24 to 48 weeks. If PCR-HCV becomes negative within 24–48 weeks, the patient is considered a responder; otherwise, drug resistance occurs [18].

As of right now, there is no effective vaccination to prevent all HCV genotypes due to the high antigenic variation and heterogeneity of the HCV genome; however, anti-HCV therapy is still developing. Additional virological and biological studies provided valuable insights into how the virus interacts with the immune system, and ultimately, this information served as a basis for designing more effective agents and led to the introduction of the development of multiple direct-acting antivirals (DAAs) [19]. By targeting the nonstructural proteins of HCV, DAAs inhibit the virus from replicating. Some types of DAAs are NS3/NS4A protease inhibitors, NS5A inhibitors, NS5B polymerase inhibitors, Cyp A inhibitors (Cyclophilin A), and Scavenger Receptor BI, such as ITX 5061. More than 95% of hepatitis C patients can be cured with DAAs; however, testing and therapy are not widely available [18].

The antiviral agents specifically target the HCV protease, which is a key player in viral replication [20]. When the protease inhibitors were combined with pegylated IFN and ribavirin, significant treatment response rates of up to 75% were reported, although this triple therapy also produced some side effects [12]. Then, several new anti-HCV drugs including ombitasvir, ledipasvir, daclatasvir, elbasvir, and velpatasvir were introduced during the following years, which target and block the HCV NS5A protein, while sofosbuvir and dasabuvir were two promising agents from the same family that they inhibited HCV NS5B protein. Initially, the combination of these drugs with pegylated IFN and ribavirin resulted in a higher SVR rate [21]. The most notable hope came when the results of a clinical trial showed that the combination of sofosbuvir and velpatasvir could produce an impressive SVR of 99% for all HCV genotypes [22]. New drug regimens were introduced as oral formulations and eliminated the need for injections. Finally, the combination of sofosbuvir/volpatasvir significantly reduced the duration of treatment to 12 weeks [23]. Another highly successful combination regimen consisting of sofosbuvir and ledipasavir resulted in SVR rates of 95–99% and reduced treatment duration to 8–12 weeks [24]. Although newer DAAs make it possible to treat HCV infections in many cases, there are still serious doubts about the 2030 goal of the World Health Organization (WHO) to eradicate

HCV [6]. One of the major problems is the diversity of the virus's outer proteins and the ability of the HCV's genomics to mutate repeatedly, making it almost impossible to develop any immunity in the host against subsequent HCV infections [25]. One of the other problems is the cost of producing and distributing anti-viral drugs, which is not possible in many countries [26]. Patients in high-risk groups face the possibility of re-infection with HCV and the need for further DAA treatment courses. Although international guidelines in HCV management do not support viral resistance tests before prescribing DAAs, the risk of developing resistant viruses in individuals and society is still serious [27]. Another point is that the development of the HCV vaccine has faced significant challenges, and it seems impossible, at least in the short term [28]. Effective DAA treatment for chronic hepatitis C patients prevents re-infection with HCV; however, high mutation rates can result in resistance to the DAAs, making an effective vaccine necessary for eradication. Also, the successful treatment does not ensure any further HCV re-infection [29].

The usage of DAA-based therapy is restricted in underdeveloped nations where treatment is most in need due to its expensive cost, serious side effects, and rapid emergence of resistance mutations. Although DAA-based therapy greatly increases SVR, finding novel therapeutic approaches that are effective for all HCV genotypes and are both clinically and financially feasible is essential. One of the novel antiviral therapies is microRNAs (miRNAs), which regulate gene expression post-transcriptionally. Because miRNAs regulate the immune system, they can either promote or inhibit the propagation of infectious diseases and are effective in diagnosis, treatment, and prognosis. miRNAs play a crucial role in cellular fate by regulating development, maturation, differentiation, apoptosis, cell signaling, interactions, and homeostasis. When HCV infection occurs, dysregulated miRNAs may either directly or indirectly affect HCV replication and/or cause liver disorders [30, 31].

1.2 The role of microRNAs in HCV co-infection

Only 2% of transcripts of the human genome are translated into proteins. Of these, over 90% are non-coding RNAs (ncRNAs), which are divided into two categories based on size: small (s)ncRNAs (less than 200 nucleotides; nt) and long (l) ncRNAs (more than 200 nt). miRNAs belong to the class of small non-coding RNAs that engage in the regulation of eukaryotic posttranscriptional genes. Mature miRNAs need to undergo many stages of processing, including: 1. The initial transcripts of the miRNA genes that RNA polymerase II controls are known as pri-miRNAs, which have a 5′ cap and 3′ poly-A tail (hairpin structure). 2. Drosha (an RNaseIII-like enzyme) and DiGeorge syndrome critical region 8 (DGCR8) cleave pri-miRNAs in the nucleus to produce the precursor miRNAs, also known as pre-miRNAs, which are 70–100 bp long. 3. Pre-miRNAs are transported to the cytoplasm by Exportin 5. They are then cleaved by Dicer to produce mature miRNA duplexes with about 22 bp of 3′-overhangs. and 4. Strand separation has been done on the only mature miRNA that can be found by its target mRNAs and enter the RNA-induced silencing complex (RISC) that contains the argonaut protein (Ago2). This string serves as a functional guide strand. The other strand is destroyed and nonfunctional [32]. The coding or 3′UTR region of the target mRNAs and the 5′ ends of the miRNA, often referred to as the "seed" region, usually interact specifically through base-paring to regulate the expression of eukaryotic genes at the post-transcriptional stage. When the target mRNA and miRNA have perfect base matching, miRNA degrades the target mRNA; if there is only partial pairing, miRNA suppresses mRNA translation (**Figure 1**) [29, 33].

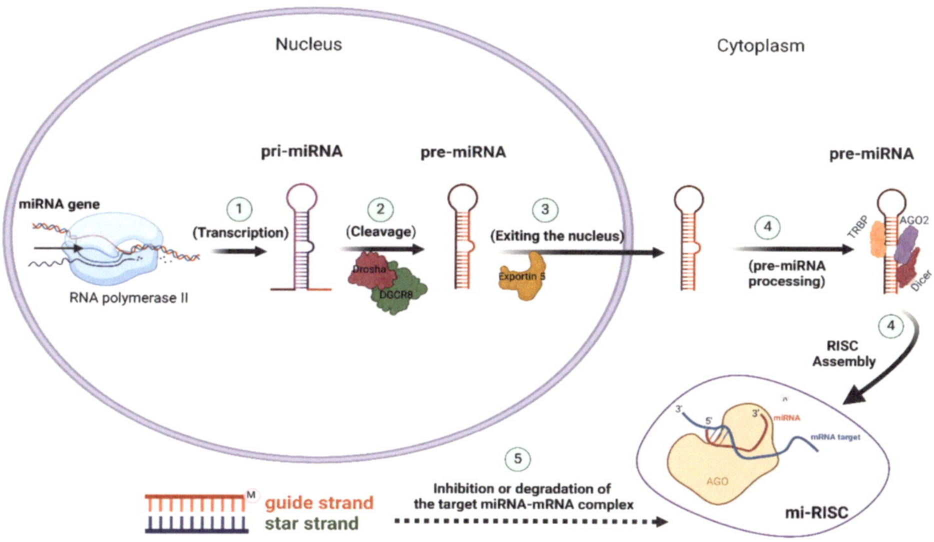

Figure 1.
The miRNA biogenesis. To sum up, a drosha-DGCR8 microprocessor processes primary-miRNA (pri-miRNA), which leads to the formation of a 70–100 nucleotide hairpin structure (precursor-miRNA, pre-miRNA). Following being transported into the cytoplasm, it matures into miRNA and is incorporated into an argonaut protein. BioRender is used to draw the figure.

It expresses over 2600 miRNAs [source: human genome database, accessed May 24, 2022; www.mirbase.org]. It is likely that multiple distinct miRNAs regulate each mRNA. MiRNAs thus appear to have a role in almost every biological function, including apoptosis, immunological response, aging, and cell division. Additionally, cellular miRNAs may influence virus replication through various interactions with viruses [34].

HCV can alter host cell functions to promote its replication, but it still needs host cells to replicate. It has been revealed that several biological factors, including miRNAs, are dysregulated during HCV infection. HCV infection modulates the expression of the cellular miRNA profile, which either directly or indirectly regulates HCV replication. Hepatocytes can alter the expression of several miRNAs to protect themselves from infection. The roles of miRNAs in HCV infection are varied. While some cellular miRNAs upregulated HCV-RNA replication (stimulation effect), others down-regulated it (inhibition effect) (**Table 1**) [36, 37].

1.2.1 Inhibition effect

Type I IFNs (IFN-α and IFN-β) intervention can quickly alter the expression of a lot of cellular miRNAs in HCV therapy. Using the analysis of cellular miRNA expression in cells stimulated with IFN β-induced miRNAs, about 30 miRNAs (miR-1, miR-30, miR-128, miR-196, miR-296, miR-351, miR-431, and miR-448) were discovered to have altered levels of expression [38]. Some studies showed that blocking these miRNAs with anti-miRNAs stopped IFN-β from killing HCV, but increasing their levels by transfecting miRNA mimics made the antiviral effect of IFN-β happen again in Huh7 cells. Apart from miRNAs that induce IFN-β synthesis, other additional miRNAs can reduce HCV replication (e.g., miR-181c, miR-199a or the Let family, like let-7b). For instance, overexpression of miR-199a inhibits HCV-RNA replication [39].

	Functions	Mechanism	References
Down-regulated microRNAs			
miR-196, miR-296, miR-351, miR-431, miR-448, miR-199a, let-7b, miR-181c	Suppressing on HCV replication	Directly interacts with the HCV genome	[29, 35]
miR-99a and miR-27a	Suppressing on HCV replication and packaging	Reducing on lipid metabolism	
miR-548 m and miR-194	Suppressing on HCV infectivity	Targeting and suppressing CD81 receptor expression	
miR-182	Suppressing on HCV infectivity	Inhibit CLDN1 expression	
miR-501-3p and miR-619-3p	Suppressing on HCV infectivity	Downregulating on OGT protein expression	
miR-29	Suppressing on HCV replication	—	
miR-185-5p	Suppressing on HCV replication	Targeting on GALNT8	
Upregulated microRNAs			
miR-122	Facilitating on HCV replication	Directly interacts with the HCV genome	
miR-141	Facilitating on HCV replication	Suppression of DLC-1 protein	
miR-134, miR-320c, miR-483-5p	Facilitating on HCV replication	Increasing of immune evasion and cell survival	
miR-491	Facilitating on HCV replication	inducing on PI3K/Akt pathway	
miR-130a, miR-373	Facilitating on HCV replication	Inhibiting on IFN pathway	

Table 1.
Some significant microRNAs were classified as either up- or down-regulated and implicated in many aspects of HCV replication at a glance.

Certain miRNAs not only directly prevent HCV-RNA replication, but they also perform so by triggering the IFN pathway. For instance, miR-130a. There have been conflicting findings from earlier research on this microRNA. It has been demonstrated that, in cells lacking TLR3 and RIG-I, such as Huh7.5.1 cells, miR-130a may indirectly suppress HCV multiplication by reestablishing the host's innate immune response. For type I IFN induction, TLR3, and RIG-I are two crucial mediators of HCC. By downregulating the expression of antiviral interferon-induced transmembrane protein 1 (IFITM1), a target protein for it, through miR-130a, HCV, on the other hand, evades the innate immune response. Since this miRNA interacts intricately with the host's innate immune system, it serves several purposes and requires further study [40].

1.2.2 Stimulation effect

Around 70% of the total miRNA present in mammalian liver tissue is liver-specific miRNA, of which miR-122 is the most prevalent liver-specific miRNA. Due to its distinct function in stimulating HCV replication rather than inhibiting it, miR-122 is an attractive target for antiviral therapies. Jopling et al. were the first to report miR-122's involvement in HCV replication. Two target sites in the 5′UTR of HCV are present in this miR-122 and are essential for HCV replication. The promotion of HCV replication essentially depends on the interaction between miR-122 and the viral 5′UTR [41, 42].

MiR-141, which HCV infection induces, may also be necessary for a robust HCV replication process. Further study is needed as the results suggest the existence of a novel mechanism of HCV infection-associated miRNA-mediated regulation of a tumor suppressor protein. Specifically, miR-141 is expressed by HCV-infected cells, and its overexpression significantly suppresses DLC-1 expression (a Rho GTPase-activating protein), mediated tumorigenic transformation [29].

1.3 The relationship between HCV and hepatocellular carcinoma

Several stages of the HCV-induced progression of HCC are associated with the viral genotype and length of the disease. Since HCV is not incorporated into the host's DNA, it is not carcinogenic. Several studies have indicated that HCV chronic infection has a significant role in the formation of HCC [43]; nevertheless, the progression of the disease and the host's immune responses are caused by HCC. Studies indicate that viral proteins are responsible for that. For example, core proteins may affect lipogenesis and oxidative stress. By altering cell signaling and cell cycling pathways and downregulating some tumor suppressor genes, such as p53 and retinoblastoma, other proteins can cause HCC [44].

Furthermore, HCV nonstructural proteins facilitate the activation of hepatic stellate cells (HSCs) and the promotion of transforming growth factor beta (TGF-β), both of which lead to liver fibrosis. Recently, studies have shown how crucial inflammation is to the growth of HCC. Some important components of hepatocarcinogenesis, such as transforming growth factors α and β, are upregulated in chronic inflammation. TGF-α upregulation causes hepatocyte dysplasia, cell regeneration, proliferation, and HCC. TGF-β is essential for inflammation in its later phases. Proliferation and differentiation processes are halted by inhibiting leukocyte activation [45, 46].

TGF-α is a strong proinflammatory cytokine that can accelerate the development of hepatocellular carcinoma and cause liver damage and cirrhosis. There is a correlation between elevated proinflammatory cytokine release and elevated TGF-α levels. As a result, several genes linked to cancer cell division, invasion, and metastasis are induced, and the proto-oncogene is activated [47].

In certain cases, untreated chronic hepatitis C (CHC) and, consequently, chronic inflammation can cause fibrosis, which can eventually progress to cirrhosis. Hepatic stellate cells and fibroblast activation happen because cirrhosis is the prelude to the majority of HCC-related HCV cases. Collagen is produced as a result. Complex structures are formed in the liver tissue as a result of an overabundance of extracellular matrix (ECM) proteins, such as collagen [48]. HSCs can synthesize collagen types IV and VI in liver injury situations. Reactive oxygen species (ROS) are produced by immune cells such as neutrophils and macrophages in response to HCV, according to certain studies. Excessive production of ROS and the inability of the body to detoxify them result in oxidative stress. It is demonstrated that HCV core protein may affect oxidative stress metabolism. Oxidative stress, which results from a disruption, is what causes liver fibrosis in the cellular redox balance. ROS activation stimulates hepatic stellate cells, turning them into myofibroblasts. These myofibroblasts produce collagen and play crucial roles in many different processes, such as inflammation, angiogenesis, regeneration, and tumorigenesis. In addition, HCV causes the dysfunction of mitochondria in hepatic cells, which is followed by the production of excessive ROS. Excessive exposure to ROS may result in abnormal signaling that promotes cell growth and survival and may play a role in the development of cancer [48, 49].

2. microRNAs: a new strategy in HCV therapy

2.1 Understanding the mechanism of microRNA in HCV

Alterations in host miRNA levels have been linked with viral infections and can influence viral infection both directly and indirectly. The genome of the *flaviviruses* includes one 3′ non-coding region (3′UTR), one 5′ non-coding region (5′UTR), and a single open reading frame (ORF). In addition to being the carrier of genetic information and having the capability of protein coding, RNAs have another important role in the regulation of the viral life cycle and its relationship with its host and vector [50]. As said before, sncRNAs are divided into small interfering RNAs (siRNAs), transfer RNA-derived small RNAs (tsRNAs), small nuclear RNAs (snRNAs), PIWI-interacting RNAs (piRNAs), vault RNAs (vtRNAs), and microRNAs (miRNAs) [51, 52]. Among them, miRNAs have been proven to affect thousands of genes. They regulate the translation of more than 60% of protein-coding genes [53] in the stable parts or tumor-associated regions of the genome [54, 55]. Compared to normal cells, miRNA expression differs in different diseases, like in hepatoma cells infected with HCV and HCC patients [56–58]. Hepatic fibrosis is followed by inflammation, which occurs as a result of the excessive accumulation of lipids in the liver [59]. During inflammation, inflammatory mediators such as TNF-α, IL-1, and IL-6 are produced by the macrophages and endothelial cells. These mediators are important for the regulation of inflammation [60, 61]. Here, we reviewed some of the miRNAs that are responsible for HCV pathogenesis (**Table 2**).

miRNA	Mechanism	References
miR-548 m	Suppression the expression of CD81	[62]
miR-99a	Decreases the intracellular lipid accumulation	[63]
miR-194	Suppression the expression of CD81	[64]
miR-501-3p and miR-619-3p	Suppresses the expression of OGT	[65]
miR-182	Suppresses the expression of CLDN1	[66]
miR-122	5′UTR of HCV interaction, Suppression the expression of OCLN	[67, 68]
miR-200c	Suppression the expression of OCLN	[69]
miR-181c	E1 and NS5A coding regions of HCV interaction	[70]
miR-196, miR-296, miR-351, miR-431 and miR-448	HCV genome interaction	[38]
let-7b	NS5B coding region and 5′-UTR of HCV interaction	[71]
miR-199a	5′UTR of HCV genome interaction	[72]
miR-21	TGF-β-mediated fibrosis enhancing	[73]
miR-141	Promote the replication of HCV	[74, 75]

Table 2.
miRNAs responsible for the HCV pathogenesis.

2.1.1 Lipid metabolism

According to the liver's function in maintaining lipid homeostasis and controlling the metabolism of triglycerides and fatty acids, infections with HCV can lead to the accumulation of fatty acids and triglycerides in the hepatic cells [76]. Several miRNAs have been reported to be responsible for the metabolism of cholesterol and fatty acids. In this era, some evidence reveals the role of miR-34a and miR-122 in sustaining the liver's metabolic homeostasis [76]. Some others that modulate the levels of cholesterol and lipids are miR-103, miR-307, miR-33, and miR-104 [77]. miR-122 account for 70% of the miRNA content of the liver, approximately is equal to more than 66,000 copies in each liver cells [59]. It is well-known for being a regulator of replication, translation, and a stabilizer of HCV through binding to the two highly conserved binding sites located in the 5′ UTR of the RNA of this virus [78, 79]. To some extent, the stimulation of translation by miR-122 occurs via the internal ribosome entry site (IRES) of HCV [80]. This miRNA stimulates lipid synthesis and storage by upregulating fatty acid and cholesterol biosynthesis enzymes, including 3-hydroxy-3-methyl-glutaryl-coenzyme A reductase (HMGCR) and fatty acid synthase (FASN) [81, 82]. In addition, miR-122 promotes lipid accumulation in HCV-infected hepatocytes. This is done by promoting the formation of lipid droplets, which leads to a suitable environment for viral replication [83]. For instance, in healthy mice, the expression of two genes encoding key enzymes related to lipogenesis has been observed to decrease following the inhibition of miR-122 [59]. On top of that, we know that HNF-4α controls different pathways in the liver that are involved in disease, such as lipid metabolism, through its effect on miR-122. In addition, it is important to know that HNF-4α controls these pathways by affecting miR-122, which is involved in a number of liver pathobiology pathways, such as lipid metabolism. Studies have demonstrated that HCV regulates these pathways through its impact on HNF-4α and subsequent modulation of miR-122 [84]. HCV uses its proteins, nonstructural proteins (NS5A) and core proteins, to downregulate the expression of HNF4α [85].

miR-34a is another miRNA that plays a crucial role in the hepatic inflammation in HCV-infected patients. This miRNA, regulates the metabolism by affecting hepatic sirtuin 1. Hepatic sirtuin 1 changes the way energy is used by turning on two proteins, the liver X receptor (LXR) and the peroxisome proliferator-activated receptor (PPAR) [86, 87]. In fact, miR-34a increases the proliferation of hepatic cells by targeting the *RXRα*, *ACSL1*, *CASP2*, and *SIRT1* genes [88, 89]. Another study reported the regulation of caspase-2 levels followed by miR-34a induction, which leads to liver steatosis in mice and humans [90]. Other miRNAs, such as miR-307, miR-33, miR-104, and miR-103, are reported to modulate cholesterol and lipid regulatory genes [77]. Some miRNAs, including miR-33a and miR-33b, are crucial to the regulatory lipid metabolism of the liver. This regulation occurs via sterol regulatory element-binding protein (SREBP) genes [91]. It has been reported that in nonalcoholic fatty-liver disease (NAFLD) patients, the inhibition of miR-34a contributes to increasing the levels of SIRT1, which results in the activation of AMP-activated protein kinase (AMPK) and PPARα and thus hepatic steatosis improvement [92].

2.1.2 Inflammation of hepatocytes

miR-155, miR-132, and miR-122 are associated with liver inflammation regarding their important roles in innate and adaptive immunity [76]. In addition to its important role in the lipid metabolism of the liver, MiR-122 has a crucial function in the inflammation of the liver. In fact, as shown by using miR-122-deficient mice, the function of this miRNA seems to be anti-inflammatory. This process is linked to the activation of the cancer-causing pathway and involves the infiltration of inflammatory cells into the liver, releasing pro-tumorigenic mediators like IL-6 and TNF. Moreover, miR-122 strongly hinders the formation of tumors [60, 61]. miR-132, which is reported to mediate inflammation and chronic liver diseases. This process has been done during malnutrition and via the enhancement of the interaction between inflammatory cells and adipocytes. miR-132 induces the progression of this interaction through the deacetylation of p65 and the inhibition of SIRT1. It is revealed that overexpression of miR-132 stimulates the production of IL-8 and MCP-1, the transfer of nuclear factor-κB (NF-κB) into the nucleus, and the acetylation of p65 [93]. Conversely, a partial decrease in the levels of IL-8 and MCP-1 and a reduction in the acetylation level of p65 are the results of the loss of miR-132. So, miR-132 inhibition may have anti-inflammatory effects in the liver [94]. It is now proven that miR-155 in viral infection regulates the innate immunity [95]. This miRNA serves as a positive regulator of inflammation. In individuals infected with HCV, miR-155 is upregulated in both the serum and monocytes [96]. Studies also suggested that some of the HCV proteins, including NS5, NS3, and the HCV core protein, have the potential to increase the production of miR-155 and TNF-α in patients with chronic HCV infection. In addition, miR-155 regulates adaptive immune responses by affecting the function and differentiation of T cells, which have a crucial role in antiviral activity. Thus, it seems that miR-155 mediates anti-inflammatory and proinflammatory signals. According to recent studies, HCV upregulates the expression of miR-155, which itself induces the secretion of TNF-α and activation of the JNK signaling pathway [97]. This phenomenon occurs through the interaction of TNF-α with TNF-R1 and recruits TRAF2, TRADD, and RIP (a serine/threonine kinase) to form a complex I, which leads to the activation of the JNK/MAPK signaling pathway [98].

2.1.3 Liver fibrosis

Liver fibrosis develops when hepatocytes are severely damaged, causing an inflammatory cytokine storm and extracellular matrix exposition. It can be caused by a number of factors, including hepatitis virus infections [99]. Some miRNAs regulate the signaling pathways, thus enabling hepatic fibrosis progression and activating hepatic stellate cells (HSCs). Activation of HSCs through multiple signaling pathways leads to severe inflammation, and it is proven that miRNAs are modulators of various growth factor receptor signals [100]. miR-29 family of miRNAs use the phosphatidylinositol 3-kinase (PI3K)/AKT signaling pathway to induce apoptosis [101–103] and thus suppress hepatic fibrosis, either by influencing collagen production and accumulation of the extracellular matrix (ECM) or by inhibiting the TGF pathway [104]. The study by Huang et al. looked at how miR-29a affected the signaling pathways of toll-like receptor 2 (TLR2) and TLR4 in cholestatic mice, which are two important factors in liver fibrosis. They reported that the overexpression of miR-29a in these mice resulted in the obstruction of the signaling of these mediators in Kupffer cells and HSCs in liver tissue [105].

miR-21, which is known as oncogenic miRNA, activates HSCs via the PTEN/AKT pathway. This pathway regulates another pathway called PI3K/AKT negatively. The modulation inhibits the activation of AKT via the dephosphorylation of phosphatidylinositol 3,4,5-trisphosphate (PIP3). AKT is located downstream of PI3K and promotes the growth, survival, and proliferation of cells when it is activated [106]. The result of one study revealed that increased miR-21 expression stimulates Krüppel-like factor 5 (KLF5) *in vitro*, which in turn promotes cancer cell migration and invasion [107]. Moreover, another study by Zhou and colleagues demonstrated that the activation of the pyruvate dehydrogenase kinase 1 (PDK1)/AKT pathway in hepatic stellate cells (HSCs) that are located near hepatocellular carcinoma (HCC), specifically cancer-associated fibroblasts, occurs by secreted exosomal miR-21 [108]. This activation occurs by targeting PTEN directly and encouraging the growth of cancer by causing angiogenic molecules to be secreted by HCC cells, including VEGF, bFGF, MMP2, MMP9, and TGF [94].

miR-221 is another miRNA that plays an important role in different cellular processes, including cell proliferation, apoptosis, and differentiation. miR-221, along with miR-222, are the most dysregulated miRNAs in the HCC case. According to studies, miR-221 is dysregulated in HCV-infected cells and upregulated in HCV-related HCC cases [109]. This happens via an NF-kB-dependent mechanism [110]. Like miR-122 and miR-222, miR-199a-5p and miR-199a-3p upregulate the liver fibrosis of HCV-infected individuals. In mouse primary stellate cells, miR-221/222 levels increased in LX-2 cells through a mechanism similar to the expression of α-smooth muscle actin mRNAs and α1(I) collagen [111].

Some of the other miRNAs related to the fibrosis of hepatic cells include miR-181b, which acts positively in the fibrosis progression through the TGF-β or NF-kB pathways. By contrast, miR-214-3p, miR-29b, and miR-101, through inhibition of the TGF pathway or suppression of collagen production in the extracellular matrix, inhibit hepatic fibrosis [104].

2.2 The potential of microRNA as a biomarker (diagnosis/prognosis) target for HCV

Since 90% of cases of liver cancer are hepatocellular carcinoma (HCC), which also happens to be the primary cause of cancer-related deaths globally, early diagnosis is crucial to improving operative treatment and patient survival [112, 113]. Given that miRNAs play a big part in the start and progression of hepatitis and hepatoma cancer and the fact that they can move from the liver to the serum through exosomes, viral particles, apoptosis, and necrosis, they have been looked at as useful and accurate biomarkers [114, 115]. One of these miRNAs that gets out of whack in cancer is miR-221. It has been studied a lot as a good biomarker for HCV diagnosis [115]. Because it plays a part in inflammation, chronic liver injury, and tumor growth, it is involved in growth, tumorigenesis, and apoptosis suppression by inhibiting the expression of SOCS3 [116], DKN1C/p57, and CDKN1B/p27 [117], as well as the activation of NF-kβ [118]. It is reported that in HCC patients, the levels of miR-221 overexpression were related to the shorter time to progression of the disease. According to the studies, the upregulation of miR-221 in the serum of people with HCC can be a non-invasive biomarker for early diagnosis. In addition, this miRNA has been demonstrated to be an independent potential predictor of tumor recurrence after resection [119]. One of the oncogenic miRNAs is miR-21, which can be used as a diagnostic biomarker regarding its important role in hepatocellular carcinoma. In a meta-analysis, the sensitivity of diagnosis using this miRNA was reported to be 85.2% (73.3–88.4%). The overall usefulness of circulating miR-21 was moderate, which indicates the possibility of using it as a biomarker for the early stages of HCC [114]. According to the role of miR-494-3p in cell proliferation, migration, and invasion, the use of this miRNA as a biomarker has been identified in some studies. In one study, the levels of miR-494-3p were reported to be significantly upregulated in HCC patients compared to other groups. These studies confirmed the potential use of this miRNA as a biomarker for HCV and HCC detection [120, 121].

Another miRNA with the role of regulating gene expression is miR-199a. An investigation related to the effect of this miRNA on HCV disease suggested the possibility of using that as a diagnostic biomarker. The reduction in the levels of miR-199a was reported repeatedly in the HCC patients [122, 123]. In addition, it is suggested that the levels of miR-199a in the serum of HCC patients may have the potential to predict the number and size of tumors in these patients [124].

Like miR-199a, miR-16 is responsible for regulating gene expression. Dysregulation of this miRNA may affect the expression of genes related to HCV infection pathways, immune response, cell cycle, and apoptosis [125]. El-Abd et al. reported that the levels of miR-16 decreased significantly in HCC patients compared to HCV patients. This reduction was more significant in patients with multiple tumors than in individuals with a single tumor [124]. miR-296, which is located in chromosome 20q, plays a crucial role in biological processes. miR296-3p and miR-296-5p are the names of mature miR-296. They drive from the 3′ arm and 5′ arm of precursor miR-296, respectively. Thus, these two miRNAs are two partners involved in tumor progression and tumorigenicity [126, 127]. The results show that high levels of miR-296-5p in the blood are linked to angiogenesis, a process that is essential for the growth of neoplasia [128]. Several studies have shown the upregulation of miR-296 both in the serum and tissue of HCC patients [129]. miRNA 486-5p is another biomarker of HCV-related HCC that is upregulated in these patients. Although the accurate mechanism has not been identified yet, it has been demonstrated that it is a highly sensitive biomarker for the diagnosis of the disease in

HCV-related HCC patients. It is also reported that the levels of this miRNA are strongly correlated with the size of the tumor and predict the invasion of the portal vein [130]. **Table 3** demonstrates other miRNAs used as biomarkers to diagnose HCV infection and related diseases.

miRNA	Expression/regulation	Etiology	Reference
miR-222	Up	HCV (diagnosis)	[131, 132]
miR-21	Up	HCV (diagnosis)	[133]
miR-99a	Down	HCV (diagnosis)	[134]
miR-122	Down	HCV (diagnosis)	[135]
miR-124	Down	HCV (diagnosis)	[136]
miR-125a-5p	Up	HCV (diagnosis)	[137]
miR-135a	Up	HCV (diagnosis)	[138]
miR-199b	Down	HCV (diagnosis)	[139]
miR-221	Up	HCV (diagnosis)	[131]
miR-122	Up	HCV (poor prognosis)	[140]
miR-148a	Up	HCV (poor prognosis)	[140]
miR-638	Down	HCV (poor prognosis)	[141]
miR-1246	Up	HCV (poor prognosis)	[140]
let-7a	Down	HCC[1]	[142, 143]
let-7b	Down	HCC	[144]
let-7c	Down	HCC	[145–147]
let-7d	Down	HCC	[142]
let-7f-1	Down	HCC	[142]
let-7 g	Down	HCC	[148–150]
miR-1	Down	HCC	[151]
miR-7	Down	HCC	[152]
miR-10a	Down	HCC	[153]
miR-10b	Down	HCC	[154]
miR-15a/16	Down	HCC	[155]
miR-15b	Down	HCC	[156]
miR-21	Down	HCC	[157]
miR-26a	Down	HCC	[158, 159]
miR-29a	Down	HCC	[160]
miR-29b	Down	HCC	[161]
miR-29c	Down	HCC	[162]
miR-31-5p	Down	HCC	[163]
miR-33b	Down	HCC	[164]
miR-34a	Down	HCC	[165, 166]
miR-98	Down	HCC	[167]

miRNA	Expression/regulation	Etiology	Reference
miR-99a	Down	HCC	[168]
miR-100	Down	HCC	[168]
miR-101	Down	HCC	[169, 170]
miR-122	Down	HCC	[171]
miR-124	Down	HCC	[172]
miR-125a	Down	HCC	[173, 174]
miR-125b	Down	HCC	[173, 175]
miR-126	Down	HCC	[176]
miR-137	Down	HCC	[177]
miR-139	Down	HCC	[132, 178]
miR-139-5p	Down	HCC	[145]
miR-140-5p	Down	HCC	[179, 180]
miR-141	Down	HCC	[75]
miR-142	Down	HCC	[181, 182]
miR-142-3p	Down	HCC	[183]
miR-144	Down	HCC	[184]
miR-145	Down	HCC	[185, 186]
miR-148a	Down	HCC	[187–189]
miR-152	Down	HCC	[190]
miR-187-3p	Down	HCC	[191]
miR-195	Down	HCC	[192, 193]
miR-194	Down	HCC	[194]
miR-199a-5p	Down	HCC	[195]
miR-200a	Down	HCC	[196]
miR-200b	Down	HCC	[145]
miR-200c	Down	HCC	[157]
miR-212	Down	HCC	[197]
miR-203	Down	HCC	[198]
miR-206	Down	HCC	[199]
miR-214	Down	HCC	[200, 201]
miR-219-5p	Down	HCC	[202]
miR-222	Down	HCC	[157]
miR-223	Down	HCC	[203]
miR-224	Down	HCC	[204]
miR-296	Down	HCC	[205]
miR-302b	Down	HCC	[206, 207]
miR-337	Down	HCC	[208]
miR-338-3p	Down	HCC	[209]
miR-340	Down	HCC	[210]

miRNA	Expression/regulation	Etiology	Reference
miR-345	Down	HCC	[211]
miR-363-3p	Down	HCC	[212]
miR-370	Down	HCC	[213]
miR-375	Down	HCC	[214, 215]
miR-376a	Down	HCC	[216]
miR-429	Down	HCC	[217]
miR-449	Down	HCC	[218]
miR-450a	Down	HCC	[219]
miR-451	Down	HCC	[220]
miR-495	Down	HCC	[221]
miR-497	Down	HCC	[222]
miR-520b/e	Down	HCC	[223, 224]
miR-539	Down	HCC	[225]
miR-612	Down	HCC	[226]
miR-637	Down	HCC	[227]
miR-10a	Up	HCC	[153, 228]
miR-10b	Up	HCC	[229]
miR-17-5p	Up	HCC	[230]
miR-18a	Up	HCC	[231]

[1]*HCC: hepatocellular carcinoma.*

Table 3.
miRNAs listing as a biomarker (diagnostic/prognosis) in HCV infection and related diseases.

2.3 The potential of microRNA as a therapeutic target for HCV

Due to the recent discoveries, there is a chance to design therapeutic mechanisms based on gene therapy for HCV and HCC-related HCV diseases. One of these mechanisms is based on using miRNAs that regulate many of these mechanisms [232]. The latest ways include host immune response modulation, direct targeting of HCV genes, liver-specific delivery to the liver (the specific cite of infection), immunomodulation and tolerance induction, and combination therapies. Although much effort and considerable progress have been made in this field, due to some problems like toxicity, many of the miRNA-based treatments have not reached clinical development [233]. Due to this circumstance, two types of miRNA drugs, including miRNA inhibitors (antagomirs) and miRNA mimics (antimirs), are trying to be developed using miRNAs [234, 235]. In other words, miRNA mimics try to treat diseases by restoring them, and antagomir corrects the patterns of miRNA expression [236]. Some examples of using miRNA as therapeutic agents in clinical trials include Miravirsen (SPC3649), which is the first miRNA used in therapeutic ways. Targeting miR-122, Roche Pharmaceuticals and Santaris Pharma are presenting it [237].

2.4 Overcoming obstacles in microRNA therapy development

Due to its high molecular weight and negative charge, miRNA delivery for therapeutic purposes faces difficulties such as limited cellular uptake, bloodstream degradation, determining the best routes of administration, controlling internal stability, focusing on particular tissues and cell types, and fast renal clearance. miRNA therapeutics use synthetic miRNAs (miRNA mimics), recombinant expression vectors, and oligonucleotide-based miRNA inhibitors (anti-miRs) to reverse pathological miRNA expression changes by enhancing or blocking suppressor and driver endogenous miRNAs. Systemic miRNA delivery faces significant obstacles in the bloodstream because of RNases' rapid degradation and renal elimination. Although systemic administration induces an immune response and causes RNA accumulation in the reticuloendothelial system (RES), chemical modifications can protect RNase digestion. Encapsulation may decrease RES absorption, prevent degradation, and extend its half-life [238].

Biocompatible, biodegradable, nonimmunogenic, stable in circulation, able to reach the target location, aid in cellular uptake, prevent lysosomal degradation, facilitate endosomal escape, and escape quickly renal clearance are all desirable qualities in a delivery system. A number of strategies, involving lipid- or polymer-based nanoparticles (e.g., chitosan and phosphatidylcholine), have been developed to successfully deliver RNAi molecules *in vivo*. The miRNA molecule is encapsulated in nanoparticle form via several delivery techniques, such as artificial expression by viral transduction, customizing therapeutic oligonucleotides by adding biomolecule conjugates or introducing chemical modifications. The nonviral miRNA delivery methods provided by nanocarriers include complexation (lipid vesicles, polymer-carriers, and gold nanoparticles), encapsulation (PLGA nanoparticles and silica nanoparticles), and conjugation; each has distinct advantages in terms of biocompatibility, specificity, targeting ability, intracellular trafficking, and miRNA release/activation processes. When you combine miRNA therapies with chemical changes, biomolecule conjugation, or carrier technology, you can make them more site-directed and effective at targeting cells. Before beginning any *in vivo* targeting, an in-depth risk assessment of miRNA treatments is necessary to reduce off-target effects and prevent miRNA overdose [239].

The following are some suggestions to overcome this treatment's obstacles [234]:

1. Small compounds developed with the use of bioinformatics innovations or chemical compound screening can be employed to get around therapy obstacles. As shown in phase II clinical trial, using the miR-122 inhibitor Miravirsen/SPC3649 (NCT01200420, NCT01872936) to overcome HCV treatment resistance can be achieved by combining miRNA-based strategies with traditional drugs.

2. A possible way to increase the therapeutic efficiency of miRNAs is by the use of amiRNAs, which are artificially generated miRNA constructs that combine siRNA sequences and miRNA primary transcript scaffolds.

3. miRNA sponges are RNA constructs that have multiple binding sites that sequester endogenous miRNAs to regulate the level of miRNAs in cells. Apart from the conventional way of administration, plant-derived miRNA-based drugs can also be taken orally; however, details regarding their absorption, function, target gene regulation, and origin in plant foods remain uncertain. To completely focus

on the therapeutic potential of miRNAs, more study is required, and dose recommendations for particular application methods are still unfulfilled.

Since miRNA therapy is still in its infancy, there is not a broad spectrum of tested carriers, and many have only been studied *in vitro* so far. In conclusion, it can be stated that there are two approaches to using miRNAs for therapeutic purposes. The first strategy involves utilizing miRNA antagonists, such as anti-miRNAs or LNAs, to suppress miRNAs that have carcinogenic qualities. Sequences complementary to endogenous miRNA are present in these oligonucleotides. Chemical changes increase their affinity for the target miRNA, and help trap the miRNA in a configuration that RISC is unable to process. These antagonists have the potential to cause endogenous miRNA degradation despite their ongoing controversy. For animal activity and cell culture, modifications that stabilize miRNA mimics and anti-miRNA to nuclease degradation and increase target RNA affinity are essential. Effective stabilizers include oligonucleotides with backbone modifications of 2′-sugar and phosphorothioate. The mentioned changes increase the binding affinity of anti-miRNA oligonucleotides to their equivalent miRNAs and confer nuclease resistance.

A second strategy makes use of miRNA replacement to make up for a tumor suppressor miRNA's lost functionality. This method introduces a fresh approach to miRNA therapy.

3. Regulatory aspects

3.1 Current clinical trials focusing on microRNA therapy in HCV

Over 60 siRNA drugs are currently in clinical trials, with two approvals, compared to less than 20 miRNA therapeutics that have not progressed to phase III trials. Endogenous miRNAs target multiple genes, but exogenous siRNAs only target specific genes. Whereas siRNAs have one to three targets, miRNAs have between 30 and 250 targets. Sequence complementarity ranges between endogenous miRNAs (30–90%) and siRNAs (100%). Consequently, a significant obstacle to the development of miRNA therapies is the diverse targets of miRNAs. To effectively use miRNA therapies, it is necessary to identify biologically significant miRNAs, regulate gene expression, and minimize nonspecific interactions [240].

Current studies for the miRNA class of their preclinical and clinical research applications as FDA-approved small RNA therapeutics start to make progress into clinical medicine. In clinical trials, miRNAs have demonstrated efficacy as miRNA therapeutics, medical intervention drugs, biomarkers, and improvements for attenuated viral vaccines [241]. Regarding this, the following two validations ought to be carried out for such treatments:

1. Preclinical validation via *in silico* analysis: before research in animal models, several of the functional roles of potential miRNAs can be assessed bioinformatically and/or *in vitro*. miRNA bioinformatics systems can simplify therapeutic candidate selection and assessment, clinical research data sources and predicting regulatory targets. Databases like ViTa (prediction of host microRNAtargets on viruses), TargetScan, miRbase, and others are available for this purpose, enhancing research efficiency. Links to most of the databases now in circulation can be found on websites like https://tools4mirs.org/ [242].

2. Validation *in vitro* and *in vivo*: cell culture platforms like primary cells, immortalized cell lines, and induced pluripotent stem (IPS) are used to evaluate the mechanisms, toxicity, and therapeutic efficacy of miRNA candidates *in vitro* and *in vivo*, supporting preclinical miRNA research and clinical trials. Clinical trials for miRNA-based therapies have been completed in the "ClinicalTrials.gov" database to date. Clinicaltrials.gov currently lacks phase III trial candidates for miRNA drugs, but early phase trials are underway to explore new candidates, including miR-122/miravirsen studies [241, 243].

Miravirsen, an LNA-based anti-miRNA ASO (15-nt LNA-PS modified ASO) developed by Santaris Pharma and Hoffman-La Roche, is currently in the clinical trial as a treatment for HCV infection, sequesters miR-122, a crucial factor for HCV replication [244]. One important miRNA for *in vivo* therapy is miRNA-122, which is involved in several physiological and pathological processes related to the liver. miR-122, which regulates HCV replication, is highly expressed in the liver. At present, phase IIa of the Miravirsen trial focuses on investigating the drug's effectiveness and long-term safety in patients suffering from persistent HCV genotype 1 infection. According to the findings, patients receiving Miravirsen did not develop any major side effects or mutations in the HCV-miR-122 RNA binding site. Effectively decreased HCV-RNA in individuals with chronic HCV genotype 1 infection (after five subcutaneous doses of Miravirsen). The reduction was dose-dependent. Miravirsen is undergoing trials and could be the first drug based on miRNA to be commercialized [245].

Mice and primates had lower liver plasma cholesterol levels when miRNA-122 was used as an antisense blockade *in vivo*. Also, binding to certain sites within the HCV-5′UTR contributes to the infection of hepatitis C. However, there is no correlation between serum levels of HCV and miRNA-122, indicating the significance of miRNA-122 in the identification of potential inhibitors [246]. Studies on this miRNA that have produced conflicting results highlight how crucial it is to manipulate miR-122 in a tissue- and time-specific approach [60, 247, 248]. According to each of these studies, depending on the cell and developmental stage, miRNA-122 levels may have highly diverse effects on a range of activities (growth, embryonic development, fibrosis, cancer development, and hepatitis C infection).

The moieties differ and include sugars, aptamers, peptides, and antibodies. To improve absorption efficiency, miRNA mimetics or inhibitors can potentially be conjugated with different moieties and then packaged into nanoparticles. miR-122, in conjunction with N-acetylgalactosamine (GalNAc), was developed to treat hepatitis C virus-infected liver (Miravirsen), with endocytosis of GalNAc-conjugated oligonucleotide drugs mediated by the asialoglycoprotein receptor. Hepatocyte cell surface asialoglycoprotein receptors are the particular binding site for GalNAc. Hepatocytes express the asialoglycoprotein receptor, enabling them to selectively absorb GalNAc-conjugated oligonucleotides. One of the main obstacles of miRNA therapy is the delivery of miRNA to the right tumor or infection site *in vivo*. To reach disease sites, miRNA mimics or inhibitors need to overcome nuclease degradation in the extracellular site. To address this problem and improve delivery efficiency, oligonucleotide modifications by chemical processes have been developed [249, 250]. miRNA-based therapy has been shown in mice, primates, and early humans to be promising for therapeutic applications. Nonetheless, complications like off-target impacts are still concerning. Since miRNAs are internal regulatory molecules, more research is necessary to fully understand their therapeutic potential [251]. Up until recently, miRNAs have been chosen as therapeutic targets due to their physiological roles and disease-specific dysregulation. For instance, in a profiling analysis conducted on a substantial group of human samples, miR-26 was initially linked to liver cancer; then, the potential of miRNA-26a was studied as an *in vivo* liver cancer treatment based on the earlier discovery demonstrating miRNA-26a downregulation in liver malignancies. Adeno-associated virus (AAV) vectors (AAVs) were used to deliver miRNA to liver cells, demonstrating tissue-dependent expression [252].

In conclusion, microRNA therapy application in public health requires a multidisciplinary strategy that takes ethical, therapeutic, legal, and scientific factors into account. To move in this direction, investments should be allocated to research and development to find microRNAs related to disease, create effective delivery techniques, and enhance the safety and efficacy profiles of treatments—the two key elements of cooperative collaboration and partnerships with regulatory bodies to set specific requirements for It demands the creation, assessment, and verification of treatments based on microRNA.

In addition to research and development, well-planned clinical trials should be carried out to assess the efficacy of microRNA therapies in various patient populations. microRNA therapy must also be integrated into the healthcare system to support therapeutic approaches and eventually clarify to patients the potential advantages as well as the risks and limitations. Finally, it is important to think about ethical issues (like getting informed consent, protecting privacy, being able to take part in research, and making sure that benefits and risks are shared equally) and cost-effectiveness (comparing the cost-effectiveness of microRNA therapy to other treatments). **Table 4** lists some microRNA-based therapies for HCV infection that have been studied in clinical trials [253].

3.2 Personalized HCV therapy with microRNA

Hepatitis-related miRNAs, which are differentially expressed in patients, are linked to pathogenesis and treatment effectiveness, with significant differences observed between patients achieving sustained virologic response (SVR) and those not. miRNAs are a viable tool for personalized medicine in the future since they can improve therapy efficacy, reduce side effects, and improve patient well-being when handled appropriately. Despite their inexperience and the need for additional research, miRNAs have a promising future in precision medicine, with major advancements predicted in the years ahead. microRNAs, a class of small non-coding RNAs, have rapidly emerged as a potential biomarker for personalized medicine, guiding physicians' clinical decisions. Personalized medicine enhances disease prediction, infection or cancer prevention, and chemoresistance by selecting effective drugs

miR-based therapeutics	Target disease	Clinical trial phases
Miravirsen (AntimiR-122)	Chronic hepatitis C (CHC)	Phase I, completed: NCT01646489 Phase II, completed: NCT01200420 Phase II, ongoing: NCT02508090
RG-101 (AntimiR-122)	Chronic hepatitis C (CHC)	Phase I, completed and Phase II, ongoing
MRX34 (miR-34 mimic)	Multiple solid tumors (HCC)	Phase I, terminated: NCT01829971

Table 4.
The list of clinical trials examining microRNA-based therapies for HCV infection.

for each patient, saving time, improving cost-effectiveness, and enhancing patient quality of life by limiting adverse effects [254].

With the beginning of FDA-approved small RNA treatments in clinical trials, recent research on miRNAs has increased their use in preclinical and clinical medicine. miRNAs can control drug resistance, treat a variety of diseases, and act as disease biomarkers for prediction, prognosis, and therapeutic agents. Since disorders of multifactorial origin currently have no effective treatments, the pleiotropic characteristics associated with non-protein-coding RNAs make them fascinating therapeutic targets. The field of diagnostic and interventional medicine is expected to continue evolving as a result of the examination of candidate miRNAs in phases III and IV of clinical research. There is potential for this unique miRNA signature to be a predictive and diagnostic tool. Physicians might then quickly and accurately diagnose diseases by matching patient profiles to databases of known miRNA signatures associated with particular diseases [255].

4. Conclusion

The possibility of novel miRNA-based therapies, diagnostics and prognostics, and vaccinations related to it is becoming notably closer as the extent of studies on miRNAs increases. miRNA-based therapies, such as miravirsen, are in phase IIb trials, indicating their potential for clinical applications. Research on the interaction between miRNA and HCV is ongoing, with the potential for manipulating miRNAs as a therapeutic option in HCV treatment still in its early stages. Identifying miRNAs involved in the HCV viral life cycle and liver disease progression opens new drug discovery frontiers against chronic HCV infections. microRNA-based therapies present a viable approach for personalized medicine and next-generation treatments by offering accuracy, efficacy, and minimal side effects in the treatment of HCV. The unique viral profiles and host characteristics of these treatments enable them to be tailored to individual patients, enhancing their potency and specificity. The use of microRNA therapy in HCV therapy provides great promise for a revolutionary change in patient care. Targeting different phases of the HCV lifecycle improves the effectiveness of antiviral medications by reducing virus replication and altering immune responses. On the other hand, issues including delivery obstacles, off-target effects, safety concerns, and an increase in viral resistance are still pressing issues that call for more research and development. Finally, as already mentioned, HCV induces liver cirrhosis to HCC in a variety of ways. Virus-induced inhibition of human tumor suppressor genes, excessive production of reactive oxygen species (ROS), and disruption of oxidative stress metabolism are a few of these strategies. Furthermore, HCV modifies these pathways by regulating the expression of miRNAs associated with proliferation and the cell cycle. Therefore, using miRNA profiles should be noticed during diagnosis and treatment.

Acknowledgements

We must first give thanks and honor to Almighty God for His favors during our search. We are grateful to dear Dr. Georgios Tsoulfas, who heads the Department of Transplantation Surgery at Aristotle University School of Medicine and is a professor of transplantation surgery. He gave us the opportunity to write and contribute a valuable chapter in the book Hepatocellular Carcinoma: A Multidisciplinary Approach about the significance of the most recent HCV treatment strategy. Dear readers, we would like to say something to each one of you. We dedicate this section of the book to the men and women who love freedom worldwide, and we sincerely thank you all.

Authors' contributions

Designing the chapter's outline (M.Sh), drafting the chapter (M.Sh, M.Z, and MR.S), collecting relevant information, and editing the initial chapter (M.Sh, M.A, and MR.S), and finalizing the chapter (M.Sh). All authors have read and agreed to the published version of this chapter.

Conflicts of interest

The authors report no conflicts of interest.

Abbreviations

AAV	adeno-associated virus (AAV) vectors
ACSL1	long-chain acyl CoA synthetase 1
AGO2	argonaute-2 protein
amiRNA	artificial microRNA
AMPK	AMP-activated protein kinase
ASO	antisense oligonucleotide
bFGF	basic fibroblast growth factor
CASP2	caspase-2 protein
CDKN1C/P57	cyclin-dependent kinase inhibitor
CHC	chronic hepatitis C
DAAs	direct-acting antivirals
DGCR8	DiGeorge syndrome critical region 8
DLC1	deleted liver cancer 1
ECM	extracellular matrix
FASN	fatty acid synthase
FDA	United States Food and Drug Administration
GalNAc	N-acetylgalactosamine
HCC	hepatocellular carcinoma
HCV	hepatitis C virus
HMGCR	hydroxy-3-methylglutaryl-coenzyme A reductase
HNF4alpha	hepatocyte nuclear factor 4alpha
HSCs	hepatic stellate cells
IFITM1	interferon-induced transmembrane protein 1
IFNs	interferons
IL	interleukin
IPS	induced pluripotent stem
IRES	internal ribosome entry site
ISRE	interferon-stimulated response element

JNK/MAPK	c-Jun N-terminal kinase/mitogen-activated protein kinases
KLF5	Krüppel-like factor 5
Lnas	locked nucleic acids
LX-2	human hepatic cell line
LXR	liver X receptor
miRNAs	microRNAs (miRs)
MMP	matrix metalloproteinases
NAFLD	nonalcoholic fatty-liver disease
ncRNA	non-coding RNA
NF-κB	nuclear factor-κB
NSP	non-structural proteins
ORF	open reading frame
OGT	O-GlcNAc transferase
OCLN	occludin protein
PCR	polymerase chain reaction
PDK	phosphoinositide-dependent kinase-1
PEG-IFN	pegylated-interferon
PI3K/AKT	phosphatidylinositol 3-kinase/protein kinase B
piRNAs	PIWI-interacting RNAs
PLGA	poly lactic-co-glycolic acid
PPAR	peroxisome proliferator-activated receptor
Pre-miRNA	precursor-miRNA
Pri-miRNA	primary-miRNA
PTEN	phosphatase and tensin protein
RES	reticuloendothelial System
RIG-1	retinoic acid-inducible gene I
RIP	receptor-interacting protein
RISC	RNA-induced silencing complex
ROS	reactive oxygen species
RXRα	retinoid X receptor α
SIR1	silent information regulator 1
siRNAs	small interfering RNAs
SIRT1	Hepatic Sirtuin 1
snRNAs	small nuclear RNAs
SOCS	suppressor of cytokine signaling
SREBP	sterol regulatory element-binding protein
SVR	sustained viral response
TGF-β	transforming growth factor-β
TLR	Toll-like receptor response
TNFR1	tumor necrosis factor receptor 1
TNF-α	tumor necrosis factor-alpha
TRADD	TNFR1-associated death domain protein
TRAF2	TNF receptor associated factor 2
TRBP	TAR RNA binding protein
tsRNAs	transfer RNA-derived small RNAs
UTR	untranslated regions
VEGF	vascular endothelial growth factor
vtRNAs	vault RNAs
WHO	World Health Organization

Author details

Maryam Shafaati[1]*, Mohammadreza Salehi[1] and Maryam Zare[2]

1 Research Center for Antibiotic Stewardship and Antimicrobial Resistance, Infectious Diseases Department, Imam Khomeini Hospital Complex, Tehran University of Medical Sciences, Tehran, Iran

2 Virology Department of Professor Alborzi Clinical Microbiology Research Center, Shiraz University of Medical Sciences, Shiraz, Iran

*Address all correspondence to: maryam.shafaati@gmail.com
and m-shafaati@farabi.tums.ac.ir

References

[1] Global Burden of Hepatitis C Working Group. Global burden of disease (GBD) for hepatitis C. The Journal of Clinical Pharmacology. 2004;**44**(1):20-29

[2] Choo QL et al. Isolation of a cDNA clone derived from a blood-borne non-A, non-B viral hepatitis genome. Science. 1989;**244**(4902):359-362

[3] Ashfaq UA et al. An overview of HCV molecular biology, replication and immune responses. Virology Journal. 2011;**8**(1):1-10

[4] Masavuli MG et al. Preclinical development and production of virus-like particles As vaccine candidates for hepatitis C. Frontiers in Microbiology. 2017;**8**:2413

[5] Zhao Z et al. Feasibility of hepatitis c elimination in China: From epidemiology, natural history, and intervention perspectives. Frontiers in Microbiology. 2022;**13**:884598

[6] Lazarus JV et al. The micro-elimination approach to eliminating hepatitis C: Strategic and operational considerations. Seminars in Liver Disease. 2018;**38**(3):181-192

[7] Smith DB et al. Expanded classification of hepatitis C virus into 7 genotypes and 67 subtypes: Updated criteria and genotype assignment web resource. Hepatology. 2014;**59**(1):318-327

[8] Tsukiyama-Kohara K, Kohara M. Hepatitis C virus: Viral quasispecies and genotypes. International Journal of Molecular Sciences. 22 Dec 2017;**19**(1):23. DOI: 10.3390/ijms19010023

[9] Hedskog C et al. Identification of 19 novel hepatitis C virus subtypes—Further expanding HCV classification. In: Open Forum Infectious Diseases. US: Oxford University Press; 2019

[10] Dusheiko G et al. Recombinant leukocyte interferon treatment of chronic hepatitis B. Hepatology. 1985;**5**(4):556-560

[11] Hoofnagle JH et al. Treatment of chronic non-A,non-B hepatitis with recombinant human alpha interferon. A preliminary report. The New England Journal of Medicine. 1986;**315**(25):1575-1578

[12] Bernal LA, Soti V. Hepatitis C virus: Insights into its history, treatment, challenges, and future directions. Cureus. 2023;**15**(8):e43924

[13] McHutchison JG et al. Interferon alfa-2b alone or in combination with ribavirin as initial treatment for chronic hepatitis C. Hepatitis interventional therapy group. The New England Journal of Medicine. 1998;**339**(21):1485-1492

[14] Reichard O et al. Ribavirin treatment for chronic hepatitis C. Lancet. 1991;**337**(8749):1058-1061

[15] Thomas E, Ghany MG, Liang TJ. The application and mechanism of action of ribavirin in therapy of hepatitis C. Antiviral Chemistry and Chemotherapy. 2012;**23**(1):1-12

[16] Pérez-Olmeda M et al. Pegylated IFN-α2b plus ribavirin as therapy for chronic hepatitis C in HIV-infected patients. AIDS. 2003;**17**(7):1023-1028

[17] Hesamizadeh K, Tavakoli A, Nikbin M. Peg-interferon plus ribavirin combination therapy in HCV mono-infected and HCV/HIV co-infected patients in Iran. Medical Journal of the Islamic Republic of Iran. 2019;**33**:63

[18] Hawsawi NM et al. Genotypes of hepatitis C virus and efficacy of direct-acting antiviral drugs among chronic hepatitis C patients in a tertiary care hospital. Tropical Medicine and Infectious Disease. 2023;**8**(2):92

[19] Das D, Pandya M. Recent advancement of direct-acting antiviral agents (DAAs) in hepatitis C therapy. Mini Reviews in Medicinal Chemistry. 2018;**18**(7):584-596

[20] Jacobson IM et al. Telaprevir for previously untreated chronic hepatitis C virus infection. The New England Journal of Medicine. 2011;**364**(25):2405-2416

[21] Poordad F et al. Ombitasvir/paritaprevir/ritonavir and dasabuvir with or without sofosbuvir for patients with hepatitis C virus genotype 1 infection who failed a prior course of direct-acting antiviral therapy. Journal of Medical Virology. 2019;**91**(7):1307-1312

[22] Feld JJ et al. Sofosbuvir and Velpatasvir for HCV genotype 1, 2, 4, 5, and 6 infection. The New England Journal of Medicine. 2015;**373**(27):2599-2607

[23] Mir F et al. Sofosbuvir/velpatasvir regimen promises an effective pan-genotypic hepatitis C virus cure. Drug Design, Development and Therapy. 2017;**11**:497-502

[24] Sulkowski MS et al. A pragmatic, randomized controlled trial of oral antivirals for the treatment of chronic hepatitis C: The PRIORITIZE study. Hepatology. 2021;**74**(6):2952-2964

[25] Wang JH et al. Characterization of antigenic variants of hepatitis C virus in immune evasion. Virology Journal. 2011;**8**:377

[26] Kaplan DE. Cost/benefit of hepatitis C treatment: It does not end with SVR. Digestive Diseases and Sciences. 2018;**63**(6):1376-1377

[27] Hayes CN et al. Road to elimination of HCV: Clinical challenges in HCV management. Liver International. 2022;**42**(9):1935-1944

[28] Duncan JD, Urbanowicz RA, Tarr AW, Ball JK. Hepatitis C virus vaccine: Challenges and prospects. Vaccines (Basel). 17 Feb 2020;**8**(1):90. DOI: 10.3390/vaccines8010090

[29] Li H-C, Yang C-H, Lo S-Y. Roles of microRNAs in hepatitis C virus replication and pathogenesis. Viruses. 2022;**14**(8):1776

[30] Jamalidoust M, Shafaati M, Kalani M, et al. MicroRNA let-7b inhibits hepatitis C virus and induces apoptosis in human hepatoma cells. Molecular Biology Reports. 2022;**49**(1):1273-1280. DOI: 10.1007/s11033-021-06955-0

[31] Shafaati M et al. Downregulation of hepatitis C virus replication by miR-196a using lentiviral vectors. Microbiology and Immunology. 2021;**65**(4):161-170

[32] Kim VN. MicroRNA biogenesis: Coordinated cropping and dicing. Nature Reviews Molecular Cell Biology. 2005;**6**(5):376-385

[33] Duan X-Q et al. The role of microRNA in hepatitis C virus replication. Journal of Clinical and Translational Hepatology. 2013;**1**(2):125

[34] Lewis BP et al. Prediction of mammalian microRNA targets. Cell. 2003;**115**(7):787-798

[35] Shrivastava S et al. MicroRNAs: Role in hepatitis C virus pathogenesis. Genes & Diseases. 2015;**2**(1):35-45

[36] Bala S, Marcos M, Szabo G. Emerging role of microRNAs in liver diseases. World Journal of Gastroenterology: WJG. 2009;**15**(45):5633

[37] Gottwein E, Cullen BR. Viral and cellular microRNAs as determinants of viral pathogenesis and immunity. Cell Host & Microbe. 2008;**3**(6):375-387

[38] Pedersen IM et al. Interferon modulation of cellular microRNAs as an antiviral mechanism. Nature. 2007;**449**(7164):919-922

[39] Pascut D et al. HCV proteins modulate the host cell miRNA expression contributing to hepatitis C pathogenesis and hepatocellular carcinoma development. Cancers. 2021;**13**(10):2485

[40] Li S et al. Micro RNA-130a inhibits HCV replication by restoring the innate immune response. Journal of Viral Hepatitis. 2014;**21**(2):121-128

[41] Esau C et al. miR-122 regulation of lipid metabolism revealed by in vivo antisense targeting. Cell Metabolism. 2006;**3**(2):87-98

[42] Li X et al. microRNAs: Novel players in hepatitis C virus infection. Clinics and Research in Hepatology and Gastroenterology. 2014;**38**(6):664-675

[43] Kanda T et al. Molecular mechanisms driving progression of liver cirrhosis towards hepatocellular carcinoma in chronic hepatitis B and C infections: A review. International Journal of Molecular Sciences. 2019;**20**(6):1358

[44] Okuda M et al. Mitochondrial injury, oxidative stress, and antioxidant gene expression are induced by hepatitis C virus core protein. Gastroenterology. 2002;**122**(2):366-375

[45] Li H et al. Hepatitis C: From inflammatory pathogenesis to anti-inflammatory/hepatoprotective therapy. World Journal of Gastroenterology. 2018;**24**(47):5297

[46] Syed V. TGF-β signaling in cancer. Journal of Cellular Biochemistry. 2016;**117**(6):1279-1287

[47] Chen H-J et al. Understanding the inflammation-cancer transformation in the development of primary liver cancer. Hepatoma Reserch. 2018;**4**(7):29

[48] Patel K, Bedossa P, Castera L. Diagnosis of liver fibrosis: Present and future. In: Seminars in Liver Disease. Vol. 35, no. 2. New York, NY: Thieme Medical Publishers; May 2015. pp. 166-183. DOI: 10.1055/s-0035-1550059. Epub 2015 May 14. PMID: 25974902

[49] Blagov A et al. The role of mitochondrial dysfunction in the development of acute and chronic hepatitis C. Frontiers in Bioscience-Scholar. 2023;**15**(3):10

[50] Ng WC et al. The 5′ and 3′ untranslated regions of the flaviviral genome. Viruses. 2017;**9**(6):137

[51] Sharma N, Singh SK. Implications of non-coding RNAs in viral infections. Reviews in Medical Virology. 2016;**26**(5):356-368

[52] Zhang X et al. The role of noncoding RNA in the transmission and pathogenicity of flaviviruses. Viruses. 2024;**16**(2):242

[53] He L, Hannon GJ. MicroRNAs: Small RNAs with a big role in gene regulation. Nature Reviews Genetics. 2004;**5**(7):522-531

[54] Garzon R et al. MicroRNA expression and function in cancer. Trends in Molecular Medicine. 2006;**12**(12):580-587

[55] Si W et al. The role and mechanisms of action of microRNAs in cancer drug resistance. Clinical Epigenetics. 2019;**11**(1):1-24

[56] Shrivastava S et al. Up-regulation of circulating miR-20a is correlated with hepatitis C virus-mediated liver disease progression. Hepatology. 2013;**58**(3):863-871

[57] Matsuura K et al. Circulating let-7 levels in plasma and extracellular vesicles correlate with hepatic fibrosis progression in chronic hepatitis C. Hepatology. 2016;**64**(3):732-745

[58] Li H, Jiang J-D, Peng Z-G. MicroRNA-mediated interactions between host and hepatitis C virus. World Journal of Gastroenterology. 2016;**22**(4):1487

[59] Jopling C. Liver-specific microRNA-122: Biogenesis and function. RNA Biology. 2012;**9**(2):137-142

[60] Hsu S-H et al. Essential metabolic, anti-inflammatory, and anti-tumorigenic functions of miR-122 in liver. The Journal of Clinical Investigation. 2012;**122**(8):2871-2883

[61] Wen J, Friedman JR. miR-122 regulates hepatic lipid metabolism and tumor suppression. The Journal of Clinical Investigation. 2012;**122**(8):2773-2776

[62] Mekky RY et al. Epigallocatechin gallate (EGCG) and miR-548m reduce HCV entry through repression of CD81 receptor in HCV cell models. Archives of Virology. 2019;**164**:1587-1595

[63] Lee EB et al. microRNA-99a restricts replication of hepatitis C virus by targeting mTOR and de novo lipogenesis. Viruses. 2020;**12**(7):696

[64] Mekky RY et al. Mir-194 is a hepatocyte gate keeper hindering HCV entry through targeting CD81 receptor. Journal of Infection. 2015;**70**(1):78-87

[65] Herzog K et al. Functional microRNA screen uncovers O-linked N-acetylglucosamine transferase as a host factor modulating hepatitis C virus morphogenesis and infectivity. Gut. 2020;**69**(2):380-392

[66] Riad SE et al. Disruption of Claudin-1 expression by miRNA-182 alters the susceptibility to viral infectivity in HCV cell models. Frontiers in Genetics. 2018;**9**:93

[67] Kunden RD et al. The role of the liver-specific microRNA, miRNA-122 in the HCV replication cycle. International Journal of Molecular Sciences. 2020;**21**(16):5677

[68] Sendi H et al. miR-122 decreases HCV entry into hepatocytes through binding to the 3′ UTR of OCLN mRNA. Liver International. 2015;**35**(4):1315-1323

[69] Elhelw DS et al. Ectopic delivery of miR-200c diminishes hepatitis C virus infectivity through transcriptional and translational repression of Occludin. Archives of Virology. 2017;**162**:3283-3291

[70] Mukherjee A et al. Transcriptional suppression of miR-181c by hepatitis C virus enhances homeobox A1 expression. Journal of Virology. 2014;**88**(14):7929-7940

[71] Cheng J-C et al. Let-7b is a novel regulator of hepatitis C virus replication. Cellular and Molecular Life Sciences. 2012;**69**:2621-2633

[72] Murakami Y et al. Regulation of the hepatitis C virus genome replication by miR-199a. Journal of Hepatology. 2009;**50**(3):453-460

[73] Marquez RT et al. Correlation between microRNA expression levels and clinical parameters associated with chronic hepatitis C viral infection in

humans. Laboratory Investigation. 2010;**90**(12):1727-1736

[74] Hayes CN, Chayama K. MicroRNAs as biomarkers for liver disease and hepatocellular carcinoma. International Journal of Molecular Sciences. 2016;**17**(3):280

[75] Banaudha K et al. MicroRNA silencing of tumor suppressor DLC-1 promotes efficient hepatitis C virus replication in primary human hepatocytes. Hepatology. 2011;**53**(1):53-61

[76] Oura K, Morishita A, Masaki T. Molecular and functional roles of microRNAs in the progression of hepatocellular carcinoma—A review. International Journal of Molecular Sciences. 2020;**21**(21):8362

[77] Rottiers V, Näär AM. MicroRNAs in metabolism and metabolic disorders. Nature Reviews Molecular Cell Biology. 2012;**13**(4):239-250

[78] Jopling CL et al. Modulation of hepatitis C virus RNA abundance by a liver-specific MicroRNA. Science. 2005;**309**(5740):1577-1581

[79] Jopling CL, Schütz S, Sarnow P. Position-dependent function for a tandem microRNA miR-122-binding site located in the hepatitis C virus RNA genome. Cell Host & Microbe. 2008;**4**(1):77-85

[80] Henke JI et al. microRNA-122 stimulates translation of hepatitis C virus RNA. The EMBO Journal. 2008;**27**(24):3300-3310

[81] Singaravelu R. Examining microRNAs as Regulators of Hepatic Lipid Homeostasis and Hepatitis C Virus Replication. [Doctoral Dissertation] Université d'Ottawa/University of Ottawa; 2016 DOI: 10.20381/ruor-5541

[82] Novák J, Olejníčková V, Tkáčová N, Santulli G. Mechanistic role of microRNAs in coupling lipid metabolism and atherosclerosis. microRNA: Basic Science: From Molecular Biology to Clinical Practice. In: Advances in Experimental Medicine and Biology. Vol. 887. New York: Springer; 2015. pp. 79-100. DOI: 10.1007/978-3-319-22380-3_5

[83] Fukuhara T, Matsuura Y. Role of miR-122 and lipid metabolism in HCV infection. Journal of Gastroenterology. 2013;**48**:169-176

[84] Wei S et al. HNF-4α regulated miR-122 contributes to development of gluconeogenesis and lipid metabolism disorders in Type 2 diabetic mice and in palmitate-treated HepG2 cells. European Journal of Pharmacology. 2016;**791**:254-263

[85] Yeh MM et al. Genomic variants link to hepatitis C racial disparities. Oncotarget. 2017;**8**(35):59455

[86] Braza-Boïls A et al. Deregulated hepatic micro RNA s underlie the association between non-alcoholic fatty liver disease and coronary artery disease. Liver International. 2016;**36**(8):1221-1229

[87] Salvoza NC et al. Association of circulating serum miR-34a and miR-122 with dyslipidemia among patients with non-alcoholic fatty liver disease. PLoS One. 2016;**11**(4):e0153497

[88] Meng F et al. Epigenetic regulation of miR-34a expression in alcoholic liver injury. The American Journal of Pathology. 2012;**181**(3):804-817

[89] Oda Y et al. Retinoid X receptor α in human liver is regulated by miR-34a. Biochemical Pharmacology. 2014;**90**(2):179-187

[90] Wan Y et al. Regulation of cellular senescence by miR-34a in alcoholic liver injury. The American Journal of Pathology. 2017;**187**(12):2788-2798

[91] Wu W-Y et al. Pterostilbene improves hepatic lipid accumulation via the MiR-34a/Sirt1/SREBP-1 pathway in fructose-fed rats. Journal of Agricultural and Food Chemistry. 2020;**68**(5):1436-1446

[92] Ding J et al. Effect of miR-34a in regulating steatosis by targeting PPARα expression in nonalcoholic fatty liver disease. Scientific Reports. 2015;**5**(1):13729

[93] Strum JC et al. MicroRNA 132 regulates nutritional stress-induced chemokine production through repression of SirT1. Molecular Endocrinology. 2009;**23**(11):1876-1884

[94] Morishita A et al. MicroRNAs in the pathogenesis of hepatocellular carcinoma: A review. Cancers. 2021;**13**(3):514

[95] Jiang M et al. Micro RNA-155 controls Toll-like receptor 3-and hepatitis C virus-induced immune responses in the liver. Journal of Viral Hepatitis. 2014;**21**(2):99-110

[96] Bala S et al. Increased microRNA-155 expression in the serum and peripheral monocytes in chronic HCV infection. Journal of Translational Medicine. 2012;**10**:1-10

[97] Zhou Y, Zhang P, Zheng X, Ye C, Li M, Bian P, et al. miR-155 regulates pro- and anti-inflammatory cytokine expression in human monocytes during chronic hepatitis C virus infection. Annals of Translational Medicine. Nov 2021;**9**(21):1618. DOI: 10.21037/atm-21-2620

[98] Trautwein C et al. Concanavalin A-induced liver cell damage: Activation of intracellular pathways triggered by tumor necrosis factor in mice. Gastroenterology. 1998;**114**(5):1035-1045

[99] Ma Z et al. Sorafenib and praziquantel synergistically attenuate Schistosoma japonicum-induced liver fibrosis in mice. Parasitology Research. 2018;**117**:2831-2839

[100] Ying HZ et al. PDGF signaling pathway in hepatic fibrosis pathogenesis and therapeutics. Molecular Medicine Reports. 2017;**16**(6):7879-7889

[101] Mann J et al. MeCP2 controls an epigenetic pathway that promotes myofibroblast transdifferentiation and fibrosis. Gastroenterology. 2010;**138**(2):705-714.e4

[102] Roderburg C et al. Micro-RNA profiling reveals a role for miR-29 in human and murine liver fibrosis. Hepatology. 2011;**53**(1):209-218

[103] Sekiya Y et al. Suppression of hepatic stellate cell activation by microRNA-29b. Biochemical and Biophysical Research Communications. 2011;**412**(1):74-79

[104] Bataller R, David A, Brenner DA. Liver fibrosis. Journal of Clinical Investigation. 2005;**115**:209-218

[105] Huang Y-H, Yang Y-L, Wang F-S. The role of miR-29a in the regulation, function, and signaling of liver fibrosis. International Journal of Molecular Sciences. 2018;**19**(7):1889

[106] Liu RH et al. Regulatory roles of microRNA-21 in fibrosis through interaction with diverse pathways. Molecular Medicine Reports. 2016;**13**(3):2359-2366

[107] Wang J et al. miR-21 promotes cell migration and invasion of hepatocellular carcinoma by targeting KLF5. Oncology Letters. 2019;**17**(2):2221-2227

[108] Zhou Y et al. Hepatocellular carcinoma-derived exosomal miRNA-21 contributes to tumor progression by converting hepatocyte stellate cells to cancer-associated fibroblasts. Journal of Experimental & Clinical Cancer Research. 2018;**37**(1):1-18

[109] Singh AK et al. Global microRNA expression profiling in the liver biopsies of hepatitis B virus–infected patients suggests specific microRNA signatures for viral persistence and hepatocellular injury. Hepatology. 2018;**67**(5):1695-1709

[110] Ding C-L et al. HCV infection induces the upregulation of miR-221 in NF-κB dependent manner. Virus Research. 2015;**196**:135-139

[111] Ogawa T et al. MicroRNA-221/222 upregulation indicates the activation of stellate cells and the progression of liver fibrosis. Gut. 2012;**61**(11):1600-1609

[112] Chen P, Zhao X, Ma L. Downregulation of microRNA-100 correlates with tumor progression and poor prognosis in hepatocellular carcinoma. Molecular and Cellular Biochemistry. 2013;**383**:49-58

[113] Shariff MI et al. Hepatocellular carcinoma: Current trends in worldwide epidemiology, risk factors, diagnosis and therapeutics. Expert Review of Gastroenterology & Hepatology. 2009;**3**(4):353-367

[114] Qu J et al. MicroRNA-21 as a diagnostic marker for hepatocellular carcinoma: A systematic review and meta-analysis. Pakistan Journal of Medical Sciences. 2019;**35**(5):1466

[115] Di Martino MT et al. miR-221/222 as biomarkers and targets for therapeutic intervention on cancer and other diseases: A systematic review. Molecular Therapy-Nucleic Acids. 2022;**27**:1191-1224

[116] Huang S et al. In vivo and in vitro effects of microRNA-221 on hepatocellular carcinoma development and progression through the JAK-STAT3 signaling pathway by targeting SOCS3. Journal of Cellular Physiology. 2019;**234**:3500. Retracted article

[117] Fornari F et al. MiR-221 controls CDKN1C/p57 and CDKN1B/p27 expression in human hepatocellular carcinoma. Oncogene. 2008;**27**(43):5651-5661

[118] Liu Z et al. miR-221 promotes growth and invasion of hepatocellular carcinoma cells by constitutive activation of NFκB. American Journal of Translational Research. 2016;**8**(11):4764

[119] Shaker O et al. miRNA-101-1 and miRNA-221 expressions and their polymorphisms as biomarkers for early diagnosis of hepatocellular carcinoma. Infection, Genetics and Evolution. 2017;**51**:173-181

[120] Li J et al. Serum microRNA expression profiling identifies serum biomarkers for HCV-related hepatocellular carcinoma. Cancer Biomarkers. 2019;**26**(4):501-512

[121] Liu K et al. miR-494 promotes cell proliferation, migration and invasion, and increased sorafenib resistance in hepatocellular carcinoma by targeting PTEN Retraction in/10.3892/or. 2021.8236. Oncology Reports. 2015;**34**(2):1003-1010

[122] Varnholt H et al. MicroRNA gene expression profile of hepatitis

C virus-associated hepatocellular carcinoma. Hepatology. 2008;**47**(4):1223-1232

[123] Jiang J et al. Association of MicroRNA expression in hepatocellular carcinomas with hepatitis infection, cirrhosis, and patient survival. Clinical Cancer Research. 2008;**14**(2):419-427

[124] El-Abd NE et al. Circulating miRNA-122, miRNA-199a, and miRNA-16 as biomarkers for early detection of hepatocellular carcinoma in Egyptian patients with chronic hepatitis C virus infection. Molecular Diagnosis & Therapy. 2015;**19**:213-220

[125] Wu W-L et al. Suppressive effects of microRNA-16 on the proliferation, invasion and metastasis of hepatocellular carcinoma cells. International Journal of Molecular Medicine. 2015;**36**(6):1713-1719

[126] Zhang Y-H et al. Prediction of microRNA-296-5p target genes and its application in lung development. Zhongguo Dang dai er ke za zhi= Chinese Journal of Contemporary Pediatrics. 2016;**18**(12):1302-1307

[127] Li H et al. MicroRNA-296: A promising target in the pathogenesis of atherosclerosis? Molecular Medicine. 2018;**24**(1):1-8

[128] Motawi TK et al. Serum microRNAs as potential biomarkers for early diagnosis of hepatitis C virus-related hepatocellular carcinoma in Egyptian patients. PLoS One. 2015;**10**(9):e0137706

[129] Su T-H et al. Serum microRNA-122 level correlates with virologic responses to pegylated interferon therapy in chronic hepatitis C. Proceedings of the National Academy of Sciences. 2013;**110**(19):7844-7849

[130] Abbasy AN et al. Role of serum micro-RNA 486-5p in Egyptian cirrhotic hepatitis C patients with hepatocellular carcinoma. The Egyptian Journal of Internal Medicine. 2024;**36**(1):1-8

[131] Karakatsanis A et al. Expression of microRNAs, miR-21, miR-31, miR-122, miR-145, miR-146a, miR-200c, miR-221, miR-222, and miR-223 in patients with hepatocellular carcinoma or intrahepatic cholangiocarcinoma and its prognostic significance. Molecular Carcinogenesis. 2013;**52**(4):297-303

[132] Wong QW et al. MiR-222 overexpression confers cell migratory advantages in hepatocellular carcinoma through enhancing AKT signaling. Clinical Cancer Research. 2010;**16**(3):867-875

[133] Wang XW, Heegaard NH, Ørum H. MicroRNAs in liver disease. Gastroenterology. 2012;**142**(7):1431-1443

[134] Li D et al. MicroRNA-99a inhibits hepatocellular carcinoma growth and correlates with prognosis of patients with hepatocellular carcinoma. Journal of Biological Chemistry. 2011;**286**(42):36677-36685

[135] Zekri A-RN et al. Serum microRNA panels as potential biomarkers for early detection of hepatocellular carcinoma on top of HCV infection. Tumor Biology. 2016;**37**:12273-12286

[136] Zheng F et al. The putative tumour suppressor microRNA-124 modulates hepatocellular carcinoma cell aggressiveness by repressing ROCK2 and EZH2. Gut. 2012;**61**(2):278-289

[137] Giray BG et al. Profiles of serum microRNAs; miR-125b-5p and miR223-3p serve as novel biomarkers for HBV-positive hepatocellular carcinoma. Molecular Biology Reports. 2014;**41**:4513-4519

[138] Liu S et al. MicroRNA-135a contributes to the development of portal vein tumor thrombus by promoting metastasis in hepatocellular carcinoma. Journal of Hepatology. 2012;**56**(2):389-396

[139] Wang C et al. Underexpressed microRNA-199b-5p targets hypoxia-inducible factor-1α in hepatocellular carcinoma and predicts prognosis of hepatocellular carcinoma patients. Journal of Gastroenterology and Hepatology. 2011;**26**(11):1630-1637

[140] Wang Y et al. Serum exosomal micro RNA s combined with alpha-fetoprotein as diagnostic markers of hepatocellular carcinoma. Cancer Medicine. 2018;**7**(5):1670-1679

[141] Shi M et al. Decreased levels of serum exosomal miR-638 predict poor prognosis in hepatocellular carcinoma. Journal of Cellular Biochemistry. 2018;**119**(6):4711-4716

[142] Wang Z et al. MYC protein inhibits transcription of the microRNA cluster MC-let-7a-1~ let-7d via noncanonical E-box. Journal of Biological Chemistry. 2011;**286**(46):39703-39714

[143] Tsang WP, Kwok TT. Let-7a microRNA suppresses therapeutics-induced cancer cell death by targeting caspase-3. Apoptosis. 2008;**13**(10):1215-1222

[144] Di Fazio P et al. Downregulation of HMGA2 by the pan-deacetylase inhibitor panobinostat is dependent on hsa-let-7b expression in liver cancer cell lines. Experimental Cell Research. 2012;**318**(15):1832-1843

[145] Au SLK et al. Enhancer of zeste homolog 2 epigenetically silences multiple tumor suppressor microRNAs to promote liver cancer metastasis. Hepatology. 2012;**56**(2):622-631

[146] Zhu X et al. Let-7c microRNA expression and clinical significance in hepatocellular carcinoma. Journal of International Medical Research. 2011;**39**(6):2323-2329

[147] Shah YM et al. Peroxisome proliferator-activated receptor α regulates a microRNA-mediated signaling cascade responsible for hepatocellular proliferation. Molecular and Cellular Biology. 2007;**27**(12):4238-4247

[148] Shimizu S et al. The let-7 family of microRNAs inhibits Bcl-xL expression and potentiates sorafenib-induced apoptosis in human hepatocellular carcinoma. Journal of Hepatology. 2010;**52**(5):698-704

[149] Ji J et al. Let-7g targets collagen type I α2 and inhibits cell migration in hepatocellular carcinoma. Journal of Hepatology. 2010;**52**(5):690-697

[150] Lan FF et al. Hsa-let-7g inhibits proliferation of hepatocellular carcinoma cells by downregulation of c-Myc and upregulation of p16INK4A. International Journal of Cancer. 2011;**128**(2):319-331

[151] Li D et al. MicroRNA-1 inhibits proliferation of hepatocarcinoma cells by targeting endothelin-1. Life Sciences. 2012;**91**(11-12):440-447

[152] Fang Y et al. MicroRNA-7 inhibits tumor growth and metastasis by targeting the phosphoinositide 3-kinase/ Akt pathway in hepatocellular carcinoma. Hepatology. 2012;**55**(6):1852-1862

[153] Yan Y et al. MicroRNA-10a is involved in the metastatic process by regulating Eph tyrosine kinase receptor A4-mediated epithelial-mesenchymal transition and adhesion in hepatoma cells. Hepatology. 2013;**57**(2):667-677

[154] Maurel M et al. A functional screening identifies five microRNAs controlling glypican-3: Role of miR-1271 down-regulation in hepatocellular carcinoma. Hepatology. 2013;**57**(1):195-204

[155] Wang Y et al. Hepatitis B viral RNA directly mediates down-regulation of the tumor suppressor microRNA miR-15a/miR-16-1 in hepatocytes. Journal of Biological Chemistry. 2013;**288**(25):18484-18493

[156] Zhang Y et al. MiR-15b mediates liver cancer cells proliferation through targeting BCL-2. International Journal of Clinical and Experimental Pathology. 2015;**8**(12):15677

[157] Ladeiro Y et al. MicroRNA profiling in hepatocellular tumors is associated with clinical features and oncogene/tumor suppressor gene mutations. Hepatology. 2008;**47**(6):1955-1963

[158] Yang X et al. MicroRNA-26a suppresses tumor growth and metastasis of human hepatocellular carcinoma by targeting interleukin-6-Stat3 pathway. Hepatology. 2013;**58**(1):158-170

[159] Kota J et al. Therapeutic microRNA delivery suppresses tumorigenesis in a murine liver cancer model. Cell. 2009;**137**(6):1005-1017

[160] Zhu X-C et al. microRNA-29a suppresses cell proliferation by targeting SPARC in hepatocellular carcinoma. International Journal of Molecular Medicine. 2012;**30**(6):1321-1326

[161] Fang JH et al. MicroRNA-29b suppresses tumor angiogenesis, invasion, and metastasis by regulating matrix metalloproteinase 2 expression. Hepatology. 2011;**54**(5):1729-1740

[162] Bae H et al. MicroRNA-29c functions as a tumor suppressor by direct targeting oncogenic SIRT1 in hepatocellular carcinoma. Oncogene. 2014;**33**(20):2557-2567

[163] Zhao G et al. Increased expression of microRNA-31-5p inhibits cell proliferation, migration, and invasion via regulating Sp1 transcription factor in HepG2 hepatocellular carcinoma cell line. Biochemical and Biophysical Research Communications. 2017;**490**(2):371-377

[164] Tian Q et al. MicroRNA-33b suppresses the proliferation and metastasis of hepatocellular carcinoma cells through the inhibition of Sal-like protein 4 expression retraction in/10.3892/ijmm.2021.5003. International Journal of Molecular Medicine. 2016;**38**(5):1587-1595

[165] Li N et al. miR-34a inhibits migration and invasion by down-regulation of c-Met expression in human hepatocellular carcinoma cells. Cancer Letters. 2009;**275**(1):44-53

[166] Yang P et al. TGF-β-miR-34a-CCL22 signaling-induced Treg cell recruitment promotes venous metastases of HBV-positive hepatocellular carcinoma. Cancer Cell. 2012;**22**(3):291-303

[167] Zhang J-J et al. miR-98 inhibits hepatocellular carcinoma cell proliferation via targeting EZH2 and suppressing Wnt/β-catenin signaling pathway. Biomedicine & Pharmacotherapy. 2017;**85**:472-478

[168] Petrelli A et al. Sequential analysis of multistage hepatocarcinogenesis reveals that miR-100 and PLK1 dysregulation is an early event maintained along tumor progression. Oncogene. 2012;**31**(42):4517-4526

[169] Wang L et al. c-Myc-mediated epigenetic silencing of MicroRNA-101 contributes to dysregulation of multiple pathways in hepatocellular carcinoma. Hepatology. 2014;**59**(5):1850-1863

[170] Li S et al. MicroRNA-101 regulates expression of the v-fos FBJ murine osteosarcoma viral oncogene homolog (FOS) oncogene in human hepatocellular carcinoma. Hepatology. 2009;**49**(4):1194-1202

[171] Reddi HV et al. The putative PAX8/PPARγ fusion oncoprotein exhibits partial tumor suppressor activity through up-regulation of micro-RNA-122 and dominant-negative PPARγ activity. Genes & Cancer. 2011;**2**(1):46-55

[172] Lang Q, Ling C. MiR-124 suppresses cell proliferation in hepatocellular carcinoma by targeting PIK3CA. Biochemical and Biophysical Research Communications. 2012;**426**(2):247-252

[173] Bi Q et al. Ectopic expression of MiR-125a inhibits the proliferation and metastasis of hepatocellular carcinoma by targeting MMP11 and VEGF. PLoS One. 2012;**7**(6):e40169

[174] Kim JK et al. Sirtuin7 oncogenic potential in human hepatocellular carcinoma and its regulation by the tumor suppressors MiR-125a-5p and MiR-125b. Hepatology. 2013;**57**(3):1055-1067

[175] Ngo-Yin Fan D et al. Histone lysine methyltransferase, suppressor of variegation 3-9 homolog 1, promotes hepatocellular carcinoma progression and is negatively regulated by microRNA-125b. Hepatology. 2013;**57**(2):637-647

[176] Jing B et al. Experimental study on the prevention of liver cancer angiogenesis via miR-126. European Review for Medical and Pharmacological Sciences. 2017;**21**(22):5096-5100

[177] Cui S et al. MicroRNA-137 has a suppressive role in liver cancer via targeting EZH2 Corrigendum in/10.3892/mmr.2018.8785 retraction in/10.3892/mmr.2022.12661. Molecular Medicine Reports. 2017;**16**(6):9494-9502

[178] Fan Q et al. Derepression of c-Fos caused by microRNA-139 down-regulation contributes to the metastasis of human hepatocellular carcinoma. Cell Biochemistry and Function. 2013;**31**(4):319-324

[179] Yang H et al. MicroRNA-140-5p suppresses tumor growth and metastasis by targeting transforming growth factor β receptor 1 and fibroblast growth factor 9 in hepatocellular carcinoma. Hepatology. 2013;**58**(1):205-217

[180] Takata A et al. MicroRNA-140 acts as a liver tumor suppressor by controlling NF-κB activity by directly targeting DNA methyltransferase 1 (Dnmt1) expression. Hepatology. 2013;**57**(1):162-170

[181] Su F et al. Over-expression of thrombospondin 4 correlates with loss of miR-142 and contributes to migration and vascular invasion of advanced hepatocellular carcinoma. Oncotarget. 2017;**8**(14):23277

[182] Yu Q et al. Loss-of-function of miR-142 by hypermethylation promotes TGF-β-mediated tumour growth and metastasis in hepatocellular carcinoma. Cell Proliferation. 2017;**50**(6):e12384

[183] Hua S et al. miR-142-3p inhibits aerobic glycolysis and cell proliferation in hepatocellular carcinoma via targeting LDHA. Biochemical and Biophysical Research Communications. 2018;**496**(3):947-954

[184] Bao H et al. MicroRNA-144 inhibits hepatocellular carcinoma cell proliferation, invasion and migration by targeting ZFX. Journal of Biosciences. 2017;**42**(1):103-111

[185] Law PT-Y et al. MiR-145 modulates multiple components of the insulin-like growth factor pathway in hepatocellular carcinoma. Carcinogenesis. 2012;**33**(6):1134-1141

[186] Jia Y et al. Tumorigenicity of cancer stem-like cells derived from hepatocarcinoma is regulated by microRNA-145. Oncology Reports. 2012;**27**(6):1865-1872

[187] Zhang J et al. MicroRNA-148a suppresses the epithelial–mesenchymal transition and metastasis of hepatoma cells by targeting met/snail signaling. Oncogene. 2014;**33**(31):4069-4076

[188] Xu X, Fan Z, Kang L, Han J, Jiang C, Zheng X, et al. Hepatitis B Virus X protein represses miRNA-148a to enhance tumorigenesis. Journal of Clinical Investigation. Feb 2013;**123**(2):630-645. DOI: 10.1172/JCI64265

[189] Gailhouste L et al. miR-148a plays a pivotal role in the liver by promoting the hepatospecific phenotype and suppressing the invasiveness of transformed cells. Hepatology. 2013;**58**(3):1153-1165

[190] Huang J et al. Down-regulated microRNA-152 induces aberrant DNA methylation in hepatitis B virus–related hepatocellular carcinoma by targeting DNA methyltransferase 1. Hepatology. 2010;**52**(1):60-70

[191] Bala S, Szabo G. MicroRNA signature in alcoholic liver disease. International Journal of Hepatology. 2012;**2012**:498232. DOI: 10.1155/2012/498232

[192] Xu T et al. MicroRNA-195 suppresses tumorigenicity and regulates G1/S transition of human hepatocellular carcinoma cells. Hepatology. 2009;**50**(1):113-121

[193] Yang X et al. MiR-195 regulates cell apoptosis of human hepatocellular carcinoma cells by targeting LATS2. Die Pharmazie-An International Journal of Pharmaceutical Sciences. 2012;**67**(7):645-651

[194] Bernal-Reyes R et al. Consenso mexicano de la enfermedad por hígado graso no alcohólico. Revista de Gastroenterología de México. 2019;**84**(1):69-99

[195] Xu N et al. Cisplatin-induced downregulation of miR-199a-5p increases drug resistance by activating autophagy in HCC cell. Biochemical and Biophysical Research Communications. 2012;**423**(4):826-831

[196] Yuan JH et al. The histone deacetylase 4/SP1/microrna-200a regulatory network contributes to aberrant histone acetylation in hepatocellular carcinoma. Hepatology. 2011;**54**(6):2025-2035

[197] Jia P et al. Upregulation of MiR-212 inhibits migration and tumorigenicity and inactivates Wnt/β-catenin signaling in human hepatocellular carcinoma. Technology in Cancer Research & Treatment. 2018;**17**:1533034618765221

[198] Wei W et al. miR-203 inhibits proliferation of HCC cells by targeting survivin. Cell Biochemistry and Function. 2013;**31**(1):82-85

[199] Zhang Y et al. microRNA-874 suppresses tumor proliferation and metastasis in hepatocellular carcinoma by targeting the DOR/EGFR/ERK pathway. Cell Death & Disease. 2018;**9**(2):130

[200] Shih T-C et al. MicroRNA-214 downregulation contributes to tumor angiogenesis by inducing secretion of the hepatoma-derived growth factor in human hepatoma. Journal of Hepatology. 2012;**57**(3):584-591

[201] Wang X et al. MiR-214 inhibits cell growth in hepatocellular carcinoma through suppression of β-catenin. Biochemical and Biophysical Research Communications. 2012;**428**(4):525-531

[202] Huang N et al. MiR-219-5p inhibits hepatocellular carcinoma cell proliferation by targeting glypican-3. FEBS Letters. 2012;**586**(6):884-891

[203] Wong QWL et al. MicroRNA-223 is commonly repressed in hepatocellular carcinoma and potentiates expression of Stathmin1. Gastroenterology. 2008;**135**(1):257-269

[204] Guichard C et al. Integrated analysis of somatic mutations and focal copy-number changes identifies key genes and pathways in hepatocellular carcinoma. Nature Genetics. 2012;**44**(6):694-698

[205] Wang L et al. miR-296 inhibits proliferation and induces apoptosis by targeting FGFR 1 in human hepatocellular carcinoma. FEBS Letters. 2016;**590**(23):4252-4262

[206] Wang L et al. miR-302b suppresses cell invasion and metastasis by directly targeting AKT2 in human hepatocellular carcinoma cells. Tumor Biology. 2016;**37**:847-855

[207] Wang L et al. MicroRNA-302b suppresses cell proliferation by targeting EGFR in human hepatocellular carcinoma SMMC-7721 cells. BMC Cancer. 2013;**13**(1):1-9

[208] Cui H et al. MicroRNA-337 regulates the PI3K/AKT and Wnt/β-catenin signaling pathways to inhibit hepatocellular carcinoma progression by targeting high-mobility group AT-hook 2. American Journal of Cancer Research. 2018;**8**(3):405

[209] Zhang T et al. Down-regulation of microRNA-338-3p promoted angiogenesis in hepatocellular carcinoma. Biomedicine & Pharmacotherapy. 2016;**84**:583-591

[210] Yuan J et al. MicroRNA-340 inhibits the proliferation and invasion of hepatocellular carcinoma cells by targeting JAK1. Biochemical and Biophysical Research Communications. 2017;**483**(1):578-584

[211] Yu M et al. miR-345 inhibits tumor metastasis and EMT by targeting IRF1-mediated mTOR/STAT3/AKT pathway in hepatocellular carcinoma. International Journal of Oncology. 2017;**50**(3):975-983

[212] Han H et al. A c-Myc-MicroRNA functional feedback loop affects hepatocarcinogenesis. Hepatology. 2013;**57**(6):2378-2389

[213] Pan XP, Wang HX, Tong DM, Li Y, Huang LH, Wang C. miRNA-370 acts as a tumor suppressor via the downregulation of PIM1 in hepatocellular carcinoma. European Review for Medical & Pharmacological Sciences. 15 Mar 2017;**21**(6):1254-1263. PMID: 28387905

[214] He X et al. MicroRNA-375 targets AEG-1 in hepatocellular carcinoma and suppresses liver cancer cell growth in vitro and in vivo. Oncogene. 2012;**31**(28):3357-3369

[215] Chang Y et al. miR-375 inhibits autophagy and reduces viability of hepatocellular carcinoma cells under hypoxic conditions. Gastroenterology. 2012;**143**(1):177-187 e8

[216] Zheng Y et al. miR-376a suppresses proliferation and induces apoptosis in hepatocellular carcinoma. FEBS Letters. 2012;**586**(16):2396-2403

[217] You X et al. Hepatitis B virus X protein upregulates oncogene Rab18 to result in the dysregulation of lipogenesis and proliferation of hepatoma cells. Carcinogenesis. 2013;**34**(7):1644-1652

[218] Buurman R et al. Histone deacetylases activate hepatocyte growth factor signaling by repressing microRNA-449 in hepatocellular carcinoma cells. Gastroenterology. 2012;**143**(3):811-820 e15

[219] Weng Z et al. microRNA-450a targets DNA methyltransferase 3a in hepatocellular carcinoma. Experimental and Therapeutic Medicine. 2011;**2**(5):951-955

[220] Liu X et al. miR-451 acts as a suppressor of angiogenesis in hepatocellular carcinoma by targeting the IL-6R-STAT3 pathway. Oncology Reports. 2016;**36**(3):1385-1392

[221] Ye Y et al. MicroRNA-495 suppresses cell proliferation and invasion of hepatocellular carcinoma by directly targeting insulin-like growth factor receptor-1 Retraction in/10.3892/etm.2022.11432. Experimental and Therapeutic Medicine. 2018;**15**(1):1150-1158

[222] Zhang M et al. miR-497 inhibits the carcinogenesis of hepatocellular carcinoma by targeting the Rictor/Akt signal pathway. International Journal of Clinical and Experimental Pathology. 2019;**12**(6):1992

[223] Zhang W et al. MicroRNA-520b inhibits growth of hepatoma cells by targeting MEKK2 and cyclin D1. PLoS One. 2012;7(2):e31450

[224] Zhang S et al. MicroRNA-520e suppresses growth of hepatoma cells by targeting the NF-κB-inducing kinase (NIK). Oncogene. 2012;**31**(31):3607-3620

[225] Liu Y et al. miR-539 inhibits FSCN1 expression and suppresses hepatocellular carcinoma migration and invasion. Oncology Reports. 2017;**37**(5):2593-2602

[226] Tao Z-H et al. miR-612 suppresses the invasive-metastatic cascade in hepatocellular carcinoma. Journal of Experimental Medicine. 2013;**210**(4):789-803

[227] Zhang JF et al. Primate-specific microRNA-637 inhibits tumorigenesis in hepatocellular carcinoma by disrupting signal transducer and activator of transcription 3 signaling. Hepatology. 2011;**54**(6):2137-2148

[228] Li Q-J et al. MicroRNA-10b promotes migration and invasion through CADM1 in human hepatocellular carcinoma cells. Tumor Biology. 2012;**33**:1455-1465

[229] Zhu Q et al. miR-10b exerts oncogenic activity in human hepatocellular carcinoma cells by targeting expression of CUB and sushi multiple domains 1 (CSMD1). BMC Cancer. 2016;**16**(1):1-10

[230] Yang F et al. miR-17-5p promotes migration of human hepatocellular carcinoma cells through the p38 mitogen-activated protein kinase-heat shock protein 27 pathway. Hepatology. 2010;**51**(5):1614-1623

[231] Liu WH et al. MicroRNA-18a prevents estrogen receptor-α expression, promoting proliferation of hepatocellular carcinoma cells. Gastroenterology. 2009;**136**(2):683-693

[232] Pan Q et al. Combined antiviral activity of interferon-α and RNA interference directed against hepatitis C without affecting vector delivery and gene silencing. Journal of Molecular Medicine. 2009;**87**:713-722

[233] Seyhan AA. Circulating microRNAs as potential biomarkers in pancreatic cancer—Advances and challenges. International Journal of Molecular Sciences. 2023;**24**(17):13340

[234] Diener C, Keller A, Meese E. Emerging concepts of miRNA therapeutics: From cells to clinic. Trends in Genetics. 2022;**38**(6):613-626

[235] Jiao LR et al. MicroRNAs targeting oncogenes are down-regulated in pancreatic malignant transformation from benign tumors. PLoS One. 2012;**7**(2):e32068

[236] Rupaimoole R, Slack FJ. MicroRNA therapeutics: Towards a new era for the management of cancer and other diseases. Nature Reviews Drug Discovery. 2017;**16**(3):203-222

[237] Gebert LF et al. Miravirsen (SPC3649) can inhibit the biogenesis of miR-122. Nucleic Acids Research. 2014;**42**(1):609-621

[238] Ben-Shushan D et al. Overcoming obstacles in microRNA delivery towards improved cancer therapy. Drug Delivery and Translational Research. 2014;**4**:38-49

[239] Momin MY et al. The challenges and opportunities in the development of MicroRNA therapeutics: A multidisciplinary viewpoint. Cells. 2021;**10**(11):3097

[240] Zhang S, Cheng Z, Wang Y, Han T. The risks of miRNA therapeutics: In a drug target perspective. Drug Design, Development and Therapy. 22 Feb 2021;**15**:721-733. DOI: 10.2147/DDDT.S288859

[241] Hanna J, Hossain GS, Kocerha J. The potential for microRNA therapeutics and clinical research. Frontiers in Genetics. 2019;**10**:478

[242] Riffo-Campos ÁL, Riquelme I, Brebi-Mieville P. Tools for sequence-based miRNA target prediction: What to choose? International Journal of Molecular Sciences. 2016;**17**(12):1987

[243] Janssen HL et al. Treatment of HCV infection by targeting microRNA. New England Journal of Medicine. 2013;**368**(18):1685-1694

[244] Drury RE, O'Connor D, Pollard AJ. The clinical application of microRNAs in infectious disease. Frontiers in Immunology. 2017;**8**:1182

[245] Chhabra R. The journey of noncoding RNA from bench to clinic. Translational Biotechnology. 1 Jan 2021;**213**:165-201. DOI: 10.1016/B978-0-12-821972-0.00016-2

[246] Lanford RE et al. Therapeutic silencing of microRNA-122 in primates with chronic hepatitis C virus infection. Science. 2010;**327**(5962):198-201

[247] Kutay H et al. Downregulation of miR-122 in the rodent and human hepatocellular carcinomas. Journal of Cellular Biochemistry. 2006;**99**(3):671-678

[248] Tsai W-C et al. MicroRNA-122 plays a critical role in liver homeostasis and hepatocarcinogenesis. The Journal of Clinical Investigation. 2012;**122**(8):2884-2897

[249] Debacker AJ et al. Delivery of oligonucleotides to the liver with

GalNAc: From research to registered therapeutic drug. Molecular Therapy. 2020;**28**(8):1759-1771

[250] Liang L, He X. A narrative review of microRNA therapeutics: Understanding the future of microRNA research. Precision Cancer Medicine. 30 Dec 2021;**33**(4). DOI: 10.21037/pcm-21-28

[251] Ishida M, Selaru FM. miRNA-based therapeutic strategies. Current Pathobiology Reports. 2013;**1**:63-70

[252] Ji J et al. MicroRNA expression, survival, and response to interferon in liver cancer. New England Journal of Medicine. 2009;**361**(15):1437-1447

[253] Monga I, Kumar M. Computational resources for prediction and analysis of functional miRNA and their targetome. In: Computational Biology of Non-Coding RNA: Methods and Protocols, Methods in Molecular Biology. Methods in Molecular Biology. Vol. 1912. New York: Springer Science+Business Media, LLC, part of Springer Nature; 2019. pp. 215-250. DOI: 10.1007/978-1-4939-8982-9_9. PMID: 30635896

[254] Condrat CE et al. miRNAs as biomarkers in disease: Latest findings regarding their role in diagnosis and prognosis. Cells. 2020;**9**(2):276

[255] Gupta S, Parveen S. Potential role of microRNAs in personalized medicine against hepatitis: A futuristic approach. Archives of Virology. 2024;**169**(2):33

Section 2

Cholangiocarcinoma

Chapter 3

Contemporary Surgical Treatment for Management of Cholangiocarcinoma

Lisa O'Kane, James V. Guarrera and Keri E. Lunsford

Abstract

Cholangiocarcinoma is the second most common cause of liver cancer and is often in advanced stages at the time of diagnosis. The disease is classified and treated by anatomic location - distal, perihilar, and intrahepatic. Diagnosis and staging workup consists of laboratory analysis including liver function, bilirubin, and tumor markers, as well as cross sectional imaging and endoscopic evaluation. Early multidisciplinary management between Hepatology, Oncology, and Surgery teams is necessary to optimize outcomes. Currently, only patients with perihilar cholangiocarcinoma are eligible for wait-list prioritization at liver transplant based on the Mayo Clinic criteria. New evidence may support the extension of eligibility for liver transplant to intrahepatic cholangiocarcinoma. As such, expanded transplant exception criteria have been proposed. Continued advances in medical and radiation therapy along with liver transplant promise to increase the treatment options and survival from patients with cholangiocarcinoma.

Keywords: cholangiocarcinoma, liver transplant, indications, diagnosis, staging, treatment, current evidence

1. Introduction

Cholangiocarcinoma (CCA) consists of malignant tumors of biliary epithelial origin that can arise from any point in the biliary tree. These tumors are classified as distal, perihilar, and intrahepatic by their anatomic location. Distal CCA (dCCA) accounts for tumors of the common bile duct from the Ampule of Vater to the insertion of the cystic duct. Perihilar CCA (pCCA) occur from the insertion of the cystic duct through the common hepatic duct and the main right and left hepatic ducts. Finally, intrahepatic CCA (iCCA) encompasses the second-order bile ducts and beyond, to the bile ductules within the liver. The histopathology of CCA also depends on the location along the biliary tree and is notoriously difficult to diagnose. Minimal or vague presenting symptoms are also typical, which decreased the frequency of early stage diagnosis. Due to this, most CCAs are diagnosed in late or advanced stages once obstructive symptoms occur, which often limits treatment options and decreases survival. Surgical resection remains the gold standard of treatment for CCA with anatomically favorable tumors in the absence of underlying liver disease; however, liver transplant can be considered for select patients with otherwise unresectable disease. In this chapter, we will discuss the histopathology, epidemiology, risk factors, diagnosis, and staging of CCA. We will focus on the surgical treatment options for CCA, especially the existing and upcoming evidence on the use of liver transplant to treat CCA.

1.1 Histopathology

Histological diagnosis has increased in complexity in recent years and now acknowledges differences in histology based on anatomic location. Overall, CCAs are adenocarcinomas arising from cholangiocytes along the epithelial lining of the biliary tract [1]. Most pCCAs and dCCAs are pure mucin producing adenocarcinoma, while most iCCAs fall into two main groups: pure mucin producing adenocarcinoma or a mixed subtype. Mixed subtype iCCA can arise from hepatocytes or cholangiocytes within the surface epithelium of the bile ducts [1]. iCCA is further classified by tumor growth pattern as mass forming, periductal-infiltrating, and intraductal growing [1, 2]. Mass forming iCCAs often display the mixed type histology and are more likely to be associated with chronic liver disease; whereas, pure mucin producing iCCA can demonstrate any growth pattern and are more commonly associated with primary sclerosing cholangitis (PSC) [1, 2]. More specific classification systems that further breakdown types of CCA do exist; however, they are not yet recognized by national and international staging systems.

1.2 Epidemiology and risk factors

Liver cancer is the third most common cause of death from cancer worldwide [3]. Of liver cancers, CCA is the second most common cause of liver cancer related mortality behind hepatocellular carcinoma, accounting for 15% of deaths [3]. Although CCA is classified as a rare cancer, the incidence is increasing worldwide, especially in East Asia [4]. In the United States, pCCA is the most common type of CCA followed by dCCA and then iCCA [2]. Worldwide, the mortality rate from iCCA has increased to 1–6/100,000 people per year, while mortality for extrahepatic CCA has decreased to less than 1/100,000 people per year [4]. The rising incidence and mortality has prompted an increase in research and development that focus on CCA treatment options, however 5-year survival from CCA remains below 20% [1].

Many of the risk factors associated with CCA are not particularly specific to the disease but more so reflect risk factors of chronic liver and biliary tract inflammation. General risk factors include alcohol use, smoking, obesity, cirrhosis, and viral hepatitis. Conditions associated with biliary stasis promote biliary inflammation, resulting in increased risk. These include choledochal cysts, cholelithiasis, choledocholithiasis, Caroli disease, and primary sclerosing cholangitis (PSC). Infection with liver flukes, predominantly found in Southeast Asia, are also considered to be a major risk factor in pathogenesis. In a recent systematic review, choledochal cysts, cholelithiasis, cirrhosis, hepatitis B, and hepatitis C were found to be the strongest risk factors for CCA worldwide [5]. By subtype, choledocholithiasis and PSC were stronger risk factors for extrahepatic CCA, while choledochal cysts, cirrhosis, and hepatitis B had greatest association with iCCA [5].

2. Diagnosis and staging

2.1 Clinical diagnosis

The presentation of patients with CCA is usually non-specific, and most patients with early-stage disease are asymptomatic. In later stages, patients usually present with vague symptoms such as weight loss, failure to thrive, malaise, and generalized abdominal pain. Large, advanced tumors can result in hepatomegaly or right upper quadrant pain due to stretch of the hepatic capsule. Biliary obstruction and jaundice can also occur and is more common in patients with perihilar and distal CCA, resulting in acholic stool, dark or "coke-colored" urine, early satiety, puritis, and cholangitis. Due to vague early symptoms, patients with CCA are usually diagnosed at later stages or as an incidental finding on workup for other illnesses; however, surveillance imaging in patients with underlying liver disease or PSC may result in earlier diagnosis.

Further investigation with a laboratory workup usually includes a complete blood count, complete metabolic panel with liver function tests and fractionated bilirubin analysis. In patients with CCA, these commonly return with a non-specific profile unless biliary obstruction is present. Based on the degree of weight loss and malaise, electrolytes and albumin abnormalities may be present. Liver function tests in the setting of concomitant liver disease or biliary obstruction may result in elevation of liver enzymes and bilirubin. Tumor markers such as carbohydrate antigen 19–9 (CA 19–9) and carcinoembryonic antigen (CEA) can be elevated in CCA, but show limitations in diagnostic sensitivity; as, CA19–9 becomes elevated in the setting of biliary obstruction. Elevated CA 19–9 at time of diagnosis of CCA has been shown to be a marker of poor prognosis and unresectability [6]. In the setting of biliary obstruction, IgG4 analysis should also be performed to rule out possible IgG4-related cholangiopathy, which can mimic CCA. In many cases, nonspecific symptoms and laboratory findings will prompt further workup with diagnostic imaging. With clinical suspicion for CCA, we recommend early referral to a center offering multidisciplinary hepatobiliary care, including a hepatobiliary surgeon and liver transplant surgeon to optimize opportunity for surgical treatment.

2.2 Diagnostic imaging and staging

Standard diagnostic imaging for CCA includes abdominal ultrasonography (US), Computed Tomography (CT), and Magnetic Resonance Imaging (MRI) including magnetic resonance cholangiopancreatography (MRCP). US is a common initial evaluation of patients with abdominal pain, especially those with biliary symptoms and jaundice. US may aid in diagnosis through evaluation of the liver, gallbladder, and pancreas. Abdominal US can detect bile duct dilation and the degree and site of obstruction with sensitivities of 89% and 94% respectively [6]. In dCCA, dilated intra and extrahepatic ducts with possible duct thickening or a discrete mass can be visible on US [7]. US findings for pCCA may include nonunion of the right and left hepatic ducts and segmental dilation [7]. In iCCA, an intrahepatic mass with irregular margins and abnormal liver echotexture is common [7]. US can also aid in staging through identification of vascular involvement [6].

Abnormal findings on US or laboratory values generally prompts cross-sectional imaging prior to specialist referral. If there is clinical suspicion for cholangiocarcinoma, we recommend contrast-enhanced CT as the next step in diagnosis and surgical planning. Triple phase CT with arterial phase (20–30 second delay post-injection), portal venous phase (60 second delay post-injection) and delayed (>3 minutes post-injection) with thin cuts through the liver, pancreas, and biliary system. A non-contrast phase is often included and can be helpful in identification of obstructing intrabiliary stones. Contrast-enhanced CT is helpful in identifying tumor anatomic location for potential resectability, tumor vascular involvement, biliary obstruction, underlying liver disease, and volumes for a potential future liver remnant (FLR) after surgical resection. On CT, iCCA is seen as a discrete liver lesion or lesions with peripheral rim enhancement on both phases, as well as contrast uptake on arterial phase and washout on venous phase [6]. Findings suggestive of pCCA on CT include left and right intrahepatic biliary ductal dilation with separation, while dCCA is associated with both intra- and extrahepatic ductular dilation, gallbladder, and common bile duct dilation [6]. Although discrete masses may not be present in pCCA or dCCA, bile duct thickening and the level of ductal dilation are suggestive of the anatomic location. Inclusion of the pelvis on CT imaging allows for the identification of peritoneal disease and drop metastases, and for this reason, we recommend inclusion of the pelvis for CT evaluation. For staging purposes, a non-contrast CT Chest is also necessary for patients with CCA. Positron emission tomography with fluorodeoxyglucose (FDG-PET) can also be used for staging purposes in patients with CCA; however, specific assessment standards are not defined. In the absence of PET avidity of the primary lesion, identification of metastatic disease with PET is limited [6].

While CT is useful in evaluation and diagnosis of CCA, MRI-MRCP offers greatest sensitivity in the identification of ductular involvement and tumor spread. We recommend combined imaging with multi-phase contrast enhanced MRI (including arterial, portal venous, and delayed phases), conventional T1 and T2 weighted sequences (including in- and out- of phase sequences), diffusion weighted imaging, and MRCP with 3D reconstructions. With this, detection of intra and extrahepatic lesions reaches almost 100% sensitivity in the assessment of bile duct obstruction [6]. MRCP is especially valuable in staging as it can precisely assess the extent of bile duct involvement, and contrast enhancement discerns vascular involvement and optimized operative planning [6]. A recent prospective study found MRI/MRCP to have a 96% diagnostic accuracy for CCA as opposed to 70% for triple phase CT [8]. Imaging characteristics of CCA on MRCP include bile duct dilation with visible stenosis and irregular thickening of the bile duct with enhancement on T2 weighted images [8].

Endoscopic retrograde cholangiopancreatography (ERCP) is commonly used to further delineate anatomy and pathology through cholangiography as well as collect specimens for tissue diagnosis. Tissue diagnosis can be made using brush cytology, direct cholangioscopic (SpyGlass) biopsy, and endoscopic ultrasound guided fine needle aspiration (FNA). In addition to brushings, FISH analysis should also be obtained to increase diagnostic sensitivity. A recent systematic review of these modalities showed the diagnostic sensitivity of FNA to be the highest at 74% [9]. ERCP can also intervene and place stents if warranted for biliary decompression. Endoscopic Ultrasound (EUS) is also widely used to evaluate lymph node status, local extent of the tumor, and vascular involvement. EUS with FNA can be used to obtain tissue samples from bile ducts and tumors along with suspicious lymph nodes. EUS with FNA is more sensitive in diagnosing pCCA and dCCA than iCCA [6].

For pCCA, it is critical that transperitoneal biopsy be avoided in any patients that might be considered a candidate for liver transplant; as, it is considered an absolute contraindication to transplant due to the risk of peritoneal seeding. This include EUS guided biopsy of the lesion or mass. EUS evaluation and FNA of any enlarged perihilar lymph nodes, on the other hand, is often required in pre-operative and pre-transplant assessment. Lymph node involvement is an absolute contraindication to liver transplant and a relative contraindication to liver resection (depending on location of the node).

Transductular biopsy of the mass with ERCP/EUS is recommended for pCCA and dCCA if possible. For iCCA, tissue biopsy is not needed to confirm diagnosis if imaging and laboratory results are characteristic [1]; however, biopsy and pathologic assessment are useful in prognostic assessment. In all cases, tumor tissue should be sent for next generation sequencing. Genetic mutation burden for CCA is high, and identification of tumor genetic mutations can assist in guiding therapy as targeted agents becomes increasingly available. At our center, we also obtain a liquid tumor biopsy for both mutation identification from circulating tumor DNA and surveillance of tumor response. A staging laparoscopy is also recommended prior to surgical intervention (either resection or transplant).

3. Current and future treatment

As previously discussed, most patients with CCA present with locally advanced or metastatic disease. Surgical resection remains the only treatment for CCA with possible cure. However, less than one third of patients are deemed resectable at time of diagnosis [10]. Even after resection, five-year survival rates remain dismal at 27–37% for dCCA, 11–41% for pCCA, and 22–44% for iCCA [10]. A multidisciplinary approach involving hepatology, medical oncology, radiation oncology, interventional gastroenterology, medical, anesthesiology, surgical oncology, and liver transplant surgery teams is necessary for every patient with CCA, and ideally treatment decisions should be guided by a multidisciplinary tumor board. In addition to resectability status, the team must ensure each patient is not only a candidate for major surgery and potentially chemotherapy but also fully optimized from a medical and nutritional stand-point.

The goal of surgery for all types of CCA is complete R0 microscopically negative resection with negative margins. Each type of CCA has different definitions of resectability and requires a unique surgical approach for resection based on anatomic locations. The decision tree for surgical options in CCA is shown in **Figure 1**. The following sections will further explore current and evolving treatment based on anatomic location.

3.1 Distal cholangiocarcinoma

Distal cholangiocarcinoma is the least common of all CCA. Resectability in dCCA is determined by local vascular involvement as well as distant metastasis. Tumor invading into the common hepatic artery, celiac axis, or superior mesenteric artery would qualify as tumor grade 4 and at least Stage 3B. Any distant metastatic disease would place it in Stage 4 and would make the disease unresectable [11]. According to the National Comprehensive Cancer Network (NCCN) guidelines, treatment would then include biliary drainage if obstruction is present, systemic chemotherapy with or without radiation, surgery, clinical trials, and palliative supportive care [12]. For unresectable disease, first line chemotherapy usually includes Durvalumab or Pembrolizumab with gemcitabine and cisplatin [12]. For resectable dCCA, upfront surgical resection with pancreaticoduodenectomy is recommended [2, 12],

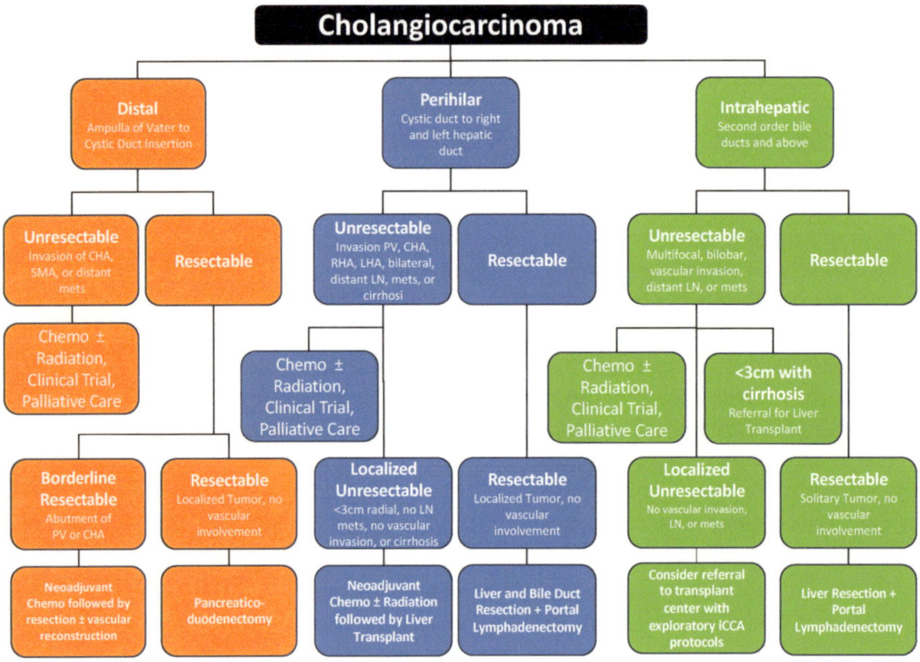

Figure 1.
Decision tree for surgical options in the treatment of cholangiocarcinoma. Abbreviations: CHA – Common Hepatic Artery; Chemo – Chemotherapy; Mets – Metastases; PV – Portal Vein; SMA – Superior Mesenteric Artery.

and neoadjuvant chemotherapy is generally reserved for patients with borderline resectable disease at presentation. After surgery, adjuvant therapy is guided by the pathologic findings. For example, if RO resection and negative lymph nodes are found then close observation is warranted [12]. If there are positive margins, aggressive pathologic characteristics, or positive lymph nodes, then adjuvant chemotherapy with Capecitabine is recommended [2, 12, 13]. Liver transplantation is not an option for patients with dCCA.

3.2 Perihilar cholangiocarcinoma

One third of patients with pCCA are resectable at presentation, however only 50% of those patients will actually be candidates for resection after staging laparoscopy due to identification of peritoneal implants [10]. Unresectability in pCCA includes tumor invasion of the main portal vein, common hepatic artery or their respective right and left branches bilaterally [11]. It also includes invasion of the second order bile ducts with involvement of the opposite side portal vein or hepatic artery [11]. Surgical resection involves the resection of the involved hepatic lobe with cholecystectomy, bile duct reconstruction, and porta hepatis lymphadenectomy [4]. Pancreaticoduodenectomy may be necessary depending on the extent of common bile duct involvement. For a resection candidate, an R0 resection is the goal, but major hepatectomy with biliary reconstruction is necessary due to the location of the tumor in the hilum. Tumor may also infiltrate microscopically beyond the visible extent of disease. In addition, the FLR must be adequate so as to not cause hepatic insufficiency after resection, which precludes patients with underlying liver disease from consideration. If the FLR is small, portal vein embolization can be done to increase the remnant size and function prior to surgery [4]. Use of neoadjuvant therapy prior to resection varies by center protocols and may be limited to patients with borderline resectability. Adjuvant chemotherapy with Capecitabine is recommended [2, 12].

Due to the potential for unresectability based on local extent or underlying liver disease, liver transplant has been explored as a surgical alternative given the increased likelihood of achieving wide negative margins. Patient selection is key, as early outcomes in patients with extensive disease were poor. The Mayo Protocol, first published in 2000, showed favorable disease-free survival and overall survival in transplant patients with small, early unresectable pCCA after neoadjuvant chemoradiation [14]. Selection for transplant requires diagnosis via positive brush cytology or intraductular biopsy for CCA, a CA 19–9 level over 100 U/mL with radiological diagnosis of malignant bile duct stricture in the absence of cholangitis, tumor extent above the cystic duct, and/or unresectability based on underlying liver disease, such as PSC [14]. In these patients, the protocol included upfront external beam radiation combined with brachytherapy and 5-fluorouracil (5-FU), with capecitabine maintenance until liver transplant [14]. Tumors less than 3 cm in radial diameter without intrahepatic, lymph node, or distant metastatic disease were considered. In this initial study, a 92% disease free survival rate at 12 months with acceptable tolerance of the chemoradiation regimen was reported [14]. Multicenter follow-up demonstrated an 82% five-year survival, and recurrence free and overall survival that exceeds that of liver resection [15, 16]. These outcomes ultimately resulted in approval of a Model of End-Stage Liver Disease (MELD) exception policy for patients with unresectable pCCA after neoadjuvant therapy by United Network of Organ Sharing (UNOS)/ Organ Procurement and Transplantation Network (OPTN) [17]. Currently, patients with unresectable pCCA who remain within selection criteria following completion of neoadjuvant chemoradiation qualify for liver transplantation listing with MELD exception [17]. Each transplant center's selection criteria must be approved by UNOS for a center to consider these patients, protocol requirements include:

1. Unresectable tumor based on location or presence of underlying liver disease.

2. Diagnosis of pCCA with malignant appearing stricture on cholangiography, positive biopsy or brush cytology, CA 19–9 greater than 100 U/mL (two of three criteria required).

3. If a mass is present then it must be less than 3 cm in radial diameter.

4. No intra or extrahepatic metastatic disease.

5. No regional lymphadenopathy or peritoneal metastasis on staging laparoscopy/ laparotomy after neoadjuvant completion.

6. No history of transperitoneal aspiration or biopsy of primary tumor due to elevated risk of tumor seeding.

Since this time, NCCN guidelines and treatment protocols consider liver transplant with neoadjuvant chemoradiation as a standard treatment for select patients with unresectable pCCA in the United States [12]. Despite adoption of these guidelines as practice standards in the United States, international acceptance of similar protocols has been limited. In 2022, a multicenter international benchmark study further investigated the outcomes between patients with pCCA qualifying for transplant compared with those who underwent resection [18]. They confirmed that among 17 international high-volume centers, patients with pCCA undergoing liver transplant had five-year overall survival of 56.3% compared with 39.9% in matched resection recipients ($p = 0.07$). Five-year recurrence-free survival was 50.2% following transplant, which was significantly better than 17.4% following resection. The overall benefit of transplant persisted in patients without underlying PSC [18]. Based on this, the authors encouraged international adaptation of liver transplant protocols for pCCA.

For patients with larger, unresectable pCCA or with regional or distant metastasis, liver transplant is not an option due to high risk of recurrent disease. Only chemoradiation, clinical trials, and supportive care are recommended [12]. Unfortunately for these patients, short term survival remains dismal even with treatment, although outcomes with medical management have improved with the advent of immunotherapy and targeted treatments. At present, down-staging is not considered in transplant protocols for patient with pCCA; however, the increased tumor response rate have been observed with recent medical therapeutic advances. In the future, reassessment of outcomes for patients with an excellent response to treatment may be warranted.

3.3 Intrahepatic cholangiocarcinoma

The incidence of iCCA has increased significantly worldwide [4]. Hepatic resection with regional lymphadenectomy to achieve negative margins is the goal of curative surgery for iCCA [12, 19]; however, less than 40% of patients with iCCA are resectable at diagnosis and five-year overall survival after resection remains low at 42% [20]. Unresectable disease includes multifocality, lymph node metastasis beyond the porta hepatis, and distant metastasis [11]. Standard treatment for locally unresectable disease includes systemic chemotherapy and/or radiation, clinical trials, and local therapy including ablation and arterially directed therapy [12].

Historically, iCCA has been considered a relative contraindication of liver transplantation due to a high instance of recurrence. Given the success of liver transplant for unresectable pCCA, increasing investigations have re-evaluated the use of transplant for unresectable iCCA. In 2004, a large retrospective study from Spain found an overall survival rate of 42% at five years for patients with unresectable iCCA after liver transplant [21]. Most included patients were only appropriately diagnosed with iCCA after explant analysis. Subsequently, a large multicenter study was conducted in Spain to further analyze outcomes of incidental or misdiagnosed tumors in patients transplanted for cirrhosis. While overall five-year survival was only 45% in these patients [22], subgroup analysis demonstrated that patients with "very early" iCCA ($\leq$ 2 cm) had superior five-year survival of 71% after liver transplant. To build on these findings, the same group conducted a larger retrospective international multicenter cohort study on patients with incidental or misdiagnosed iCCA found on the explants following transplant for HCC or cirrhosis [23]. The cohort was similarly divided into very early iCCA ($\leq$ 2 cm) and advanced iCCA (>2 cm or multifocal). Risk of recurrence at five years was 18% in the very early group compared to 61% in the advanced group. Five-year overall survival was similarly improved at 65% in the very early group versus 45% in the advanced group.

While outcomes for liver transplant with small, solitary iCCA in a background of cirrhosis showed promise, the strict inclusion criteria severely limits patients who might benefit from implementation of such a protocol. A multi-center cohort of French Transplant centers subsequently performed retrospective analysis of patients with incidentally diagnosed iCCA or mixed iCCA/HCC after liver transplant for patients with a cumulative tumor diameter of 2–5 cm compared to liver resection [24]. Liver transplant recipients with tumors >2 cm but ≤5 cm had 5-year recurrence of 21% compared with 48% for liver resection, and 5-year recurrence free survival was 75% for liver transplant compared with 36% for liver resection. Furthermore, on multivariate assessment, liver transplant was protective against recurrence (HR 0.23, 95% CI 0.07–0.82, $p = 0.02$), while independent predictors of recurrence included diameter of the largest nodule (HR 1.10, 95% CI 1.02–1.73, $p = 0.007$) and differentiation (HR 4.16, 95% CI 1.37–12.66, $p = 0.01$). Overall survival for liver transplant recipients with tumors 2-5 cm was 65% at 5 years. While this series only included 49 patients undergoing liver transplant, acceptable survival outcomes may be achieved with expansion of size restrictions beyond 2 cm. These results also supported the need for prospective trials to better assess the candidacy of patients with early iCCA and cirrhosis for transplantation. Support for consideration for transplant candidacy in patients with small iCCA on a background of cirrhosis has subsequently grown, and MELD exception for patients with iCCA ≤3 cm in the setting of underlying cirrhosis has recently been proposed by UNOS/OPTN [25].

While support for transplant for early iCCA in the setting of cirrhosis has increased, limited data was available regarding the efficacy of liver transplant for larger, unresectable, liver-limited iCCA in the absence of underlying liver disease. In 2018, a small prospective case series was conducted by Houston Methodist Hospital and MD Anderson Cancer Center on liver transplant for locally advanced, unresectable iCCA after gemcitabine based neoadjuvant chemotherapy [26]. Under this protocol, six months disease stability or response to therapy rather than tumor size were used as patient selection criteria for transplant. Although only six patients received transplantation, the overall survival was 83.3% with 50% recurrence free survival at five years. Continuing this protocol, this group subsequently reported a follow-up series of 18 patients receiving liver transplant [27]. Overall survival was 57% at five-years survival with 38% disease recurrence, with multifocality increasing the risk of recurrent disease. In intent to treat analysis, qualifying patients that did not receive transplant had 100% mortality at two years. Although these protocols provide insight and possible favorable outcomes of liver transplant for patients with iCCA, additional prospective data is needed to support this indication. At this time, liver transplant for larger iCCA remains restricted to research protocols, but consideration for referral to a transplant center evaluating such protocols should be considered.

4. Conclusion

CCA remains a rare and deadly disease. However, the incidence of liver disease and liver cancer including CCA are increasing worldwide. Managing risk factors and comorbidities is an important step to decrease the disease presence but once CCA is diagnosed survival is poor. Medical and surgical advances are attempting to combat this deadly disease with improved early diagnosis as well as more effective chemotherapy, chemoradiation, localized therapies, and surgical intervention. Although surgical resection remains the gold standard in treatment for all types of CCA, liver transplantation offers a promising avenue for select patient with either pCCA or iCCA. Additional developments in neoadjuvant chemoradiation may beneficially impact future surgical outcomes in resection and transplantation.

Conflict of interest

The authors declare no conflict of interest.

Notes/thanks/other declarations

"The views and information presented are those of the authors and do not represent the official position of the U.S. Army Medical Center of Excellence, the U.S. Army Training and Doctrine Command, or the Departments of Army, Department of Defense, or U.S. Government."

Author details

Lisa O'Kane[1*], James V. Guarrera[2] and Keri E. Lunsford[2,3]

1 Department of Surgery, St. Joseph's University Medical Center, Paterson, NJ, USA

2 Department of Surgery, Division of Transplant and Hepatobiliary Surgery, Rutgers New Jersey Medical School, Newark, NJ, USA

3 Center for Immunity and Inflammation, Rutgers New Jersey Medical School, Newark, NJ, USA

*Address all correspondence to: lokane5@gmail.com

References

[1] Banales JM, Marin JJG, Lamarca A, et al. Cholangiocarcinoma 2020: The next horizon in mechanisms and management. Nature Reviews. Gastroenterology and Hepatology. 2020;**17**:557-588

[2] Banales JM, Cardinale V, Carpino G, et al. Cholangiocarcinoma: Current knowledge and future perspectives consensus statement from the European network for the study of Cholangiocarcinoma (ENS-CCA). Nature Reviews Gastroenterology and Hepatology. 2016;**13**:261-280

[3] Rumgay H, Ferlay J, de Martel C, et al. Global, regional, and national burden of primary liver cancer by subtype. European Journal of Cancer. 2022;**161**:108-118

[4] Bertuccio P, Malvezzi M, Cariolo G, et al. Global trends in mortality from intrahepatic and extrahepatic cholangiocarcinoma. Journal of Hepatology. 2019;**71**(1):104-114

[5] Clements O, Eliahoo J, Kim JU, Taylor-Robinson SD, Khan SA. Risk factors for intrahepatic and extrahepatic cholangiocarcinoma: A systematic review and meta-analysis. Journal of Hepatology. 2020;**72**(1):95-103

[6] Shin DW, Moon SH, Kim JH. Diagnosis of Cholangiocarcinoma. Diagnostics. 2023;**13**(233):1-14

[7] Bloom CM, Langer B, Wilson SR. Role of US in the detection, characterization, and staging of cholangiocarcinoma. Radio Graphics. 1999;**19**(5):1199-1218

[8] Ke C, Yang T, Huang G, Gu C. Investigation of the accuracy of magnetic resonance cholangiography and multi-slice spiral computed tomography in the diagnosis of cholangiocarcinoma. Journal of Gastrointestinal Oncology. 2023;**14**(3):1496-1503

[9] Yoon SB, Moon SH, Ko SW, et al. Brush cytology, forceps biopsy, or endoscopic ultrasound guided sampling for diagnosis of bile duct cancer: A meta-analysis. Digestive Diseases and Sciences. 2022;**67**:3284-3297

[10] Khan SA, Davidson BR, Goldin RD, et al. Guidelines for the diagnosis and treatment of Cholangiocarcinoma: An update. Gut. 2012;**61**:1657-1669

[11] Edge SB, Greene FL, Schilsky RL, et al. American Joint Cancer Committee (AJCC) Cancer Staging Manual. 8th ed. Chicago, Illinois, USA: The American College of Surgeons; Springer Nature. 2017

[12] National Comprehensive Cancer Network Guidelines Version 2.2024. Biliary Tract Cancers

[13] Primrose JN, Fox RP, Palmer DH, et al. Capecitabine compared with observation in resected biliary tract cancer (BILCAP): A randomized, controlled, multicenter, phase 3 study. The Lancet Oncology. 2019;**20**:663-673

[14] De Vreede I, Steers JL, Burch PA, et al. Prolonged disease-free survival after orthotopic liver transplantation plus adjuvant chemoirradiation for cholangiocarcinoma. Liver Transplantation. 2000;**6**(3):309-316

[15] Heimbach JK, Gores GJ, Haddock MG, et al. Liver transplantation for unresectable perihilar cholangiocarcinoma. Seminars in Liver Disease. 2004;**24**(2):201-207

[16] Rea DJ, Heimbach JK, Rosen CB, et al. Liver transplantation with neoadjuvant chemoradiation is more effective than resection for hilar cholangiocarcinoma. Annals of Surgery. 2005;**242**(3):451-458

[17] Gores GJ, Gish RG, Sudan D, Rosen CB, The MELD Exception Study Group. Model for end-stage liver disease (MELD) exception for cholangiocarcinoma or biliary dysplasia. Liver Transplantation. 2006;**12**:95-97

[18] Breuer E, Mueller M, Doyle MB, et al. Liver transplantation as a new standard of care in patients with perihilar cholangiocarcinoma? Results from an international benchmark study. Annals of Surgery. 2022;**276**(5):846-853

[19] Bowlus CL, Arrive L, Bergquist A, et al. AASLD practice guidance on primary sclerosing cholangitis and cholangiocarcinoma. Hepatology. 2023;**77**:659-702

[20] Tan JCC, Coburn NG, Baxter NN, Kiss A, Law CHL. Surgical management of intrahepatic cholangiocarcinoma-a population-based study. Annals of Surgical Oncology. 2008;**15**(2):600-608

[21] Robles R, Figuera J, Turrion VS, et al. Spanish experience with liver transplantation for hilar and peripheral cholangiocarcinoma. Annals of Surgery. 2004;**239**:265-271

[22] Sapisochin G, Rodriguez de Lope C, Gastaca M, et al. "Very early" intrahepatic cholangiocarcinoma in cirrhotic patient: Should liver transplantation be reconsidered in these patients? American Journal of Transplantation. 2014;**14**:660-667

[23] Sapisochin G, Facciuto M, Rubbia-Brandt L, et al. Liver transplantation for "very early" intrahepatic cholangiocarcinoma: International retrospective study supporting a prospective assessment. Hepatology. 2016;**64**(4):1178-1188

[24] De Martin E, Rayar M, Golse N, et al. Analysis of liver resection versus liver transplantation on outcome of small intrahepatic Cholangiocarcinoma and combined hepatocellular-Cholangiocarcinoma in the setting of cirrhosis. Liver Transplantation. 2020;**26**(6):785-798

[25] Liver and Intestinal Organ Transplantation Committee. National Liver Review Board (NLRB) Updates Related to Transplant Oncology. USA: Organ Procurement and Transplant Network (OPTN); 2024

[26] Lunsford KE, Javle M, Heyne K, et al. Liver transplantation for locally advanced intrahepatic cholangiocarcinoma treated with neoadjuvant therapy: A prospective case-series. The Lancet Gastroenterology and Hepatology. 2018;**3**(5):337-348

[27] McMillan RR, Javle M, Kodali S, et al. Survival following liver transplantation for locally advanced, unresectable intrahepatic cholangiocarcinoma. American Journal of Transplantation. 2022;**22**(3):823-832

Section 3

Hepatocellular Carcinoma

Chapter 4

Hepatocellular Carcinoma: Locoregional Therapies and Multidisciplinary Strategies

Ioannis Margaris, Nikolaos Arkadopoulos and Ioannis Hatzaras

Abstract

Hepatocellular carcinoma (HCC) is an increasingly common malignancy worldwide. Transarterial chemoembolization (TACE) is a procedure that was developed to treat HCC patients deemed unsuitable candidates for surgical resection or transplantation and has shown a survival benefit for patients with unresectable HCC. Similarly, radiofrequency ablation (RFA) and microwave ablation (MWA) have been shown to treat HCC successfully, although the rates of success are size-dependent. Head-to-head studies of TACE vs. RFA have shown some superiority of ablation vs. TACE in prolonging survival, with the greatest survival benefit conferred to individuals undergoing dual TACE and ablation therapy. The chapter will discuss the merits of combination treatment vs. monotherapy.

Keywords: ablation, chemoembolization, monotherapy, combination treatment, prognosis, hepatocellular carcinoma

1. Introduction

Hepatocellular carcinoma (HCC) is the most common primary liver tumor worldwide and a major component of cancer-related mortality. It is a major health concern worldwide, particularly in regions with high rates of hepatitis B and C infections. Surgical treatment, including either liver resection or liver transplantation, has long been considered the standard of care for early hepatocellular carcinoma; when applied in carefully selected patients, it can offer five-year survival rates in the range of 60–80% with minimal postoperative morbidity and mortality. When planning a surgical resection, tumor size, multifocality, liver function, and patients' performance status should all be taken into account. Liver transplantation has consistently been the treatment strategy leading to the highest cure rates. It combines treatment of both the malignant tumor and the underlying cirrhosis. Traditional indications include the presence of tumor not amenable to resection but within the Milan criteria. Furthermore, patients initially beyond the Milan criteria can ultimately be considered for transplantation after downstaging within appropriate protocols.

Advances in the field of surgery and continuous refinements of surgical techniques, along with breakthroughs in locoregional therapies and systematic therapies, have paved the way toward a multidisciplinary and individualized approach in treating patients with HCC. Treatment allocation commonly follows the Barcelona Clinic Liver Cancer (BCLC) staging system, which not only provides prognostic information but also makes treatment recommendations by integrating factors such as tumor status, liver function, and health status. According to that rather simplified but non-exhaustive scheme, ablative techniques are indicated for very early and early-stage HCC (*stage 0-A*), while chemoembolization is the standard treatment applied in intermediate-stage HCC (*stage B*). Advanced disease stage (*stage C*) calls for systematic treatment. We herein discuss the most widely used locoregional techniques, as well as a combination of multidisciplinary strategies that can benefit especially the patient who is not a resection nor a transplantation candidate.

2. Local ablation

Ablation therapy for HCC is a minimally invasive treatment aimed at destroying cancer cells within the liver. It is particularly effective for small, localized tumors and offers several advantages, including preserving healthy liver tissue and providing a curative option for patients who are not candidates for surgery or liver transplantation. Advantages include a minimally invasive procedure with reduced recovery time compared to surgery, which is often performed in the outpatient setting with local anesthesia and some sedation. This procedure can be repeated if new tumors develop, and they tend to preserve more healthy liver tissue. Disadvantages include a modality that is in general limited to smaller tumors, as there is a risk of incomplete ablation or recurrence, particularly with larger or poorly defined tumors.

The broad category of local ablation includes hyperthermic techniques, such as radiofrequency ablation (RFA) and microwave ablation (MWA), cryoablation (which is based on the cooling effect), and non-thermal techniques (percutaneous ethanol injection and irreversible electroporation).

Radiofrequency ablation (RFA) is perhaps the most widely used ablative treatment for hepatocellular carcinoma (HCC), especially for patients with small, localized tumors who are not candidates for surgical resection or liver transplantation. RFA uses high-frequency electrical currents to generate heat, which destroys cancer cells. The mechanism of action for RFA involves the use of an electrode probe (which may be a needle-like probe with multiple prongs) that is inserted into the tumor under imaging guidance (usually ultrasound). High-frequency electrical currents pass through the probe, creating thermal energy that heats the tumor tissue to temperatures of 60–100°C, resulting in coagulative necrosis of cancer cells.

Thermal Coagulation occurs when the generated heat increases the temperature of the tumor tissue to between 60 and 100°C. At these temperatures, protein denaturation and coagulative necrosis occur. The high temperatures induce cell death by protein denaturation (proteins within the cancer cells are denatured and lose their functional and structural integrity), cell membrane disruption (the heat damages cell membranes, causing loss of cell homeostasis and subsequent cell death) and ultimately coagulative necrosis (cells die alas retain their architectural outline for some time before being resorbed local macrophages).

Possible limitations include: increasing size of the tumor, neighboring vascular structures, and inaccessible location of the tumor within the hepatic parenchyma. In general, a tumor threshold of 2 cm defines optimal results with RFA; efficacy is reduced beyond that limit, likely because malignant microsatellites are more frequent with larger tumors. Lesions in proximity to large vascular structures may also reduce the efficacy of RFA, due to a phenomenon called "heat-sink" effect, which transfers heat energy toward the blood flow and might, therefore, reduce the size of the thermal ablation zone. Lastly, tumor locations close to the gallbladder or concealed by adhesions (e.g., due to previous laparotomies) or bowel loops may render the technique unfeasible. Currently, RFA is considered the treatment of choice for single tumors less than 2 cm in favorable locations and patients with preserved liver function and good performance status (very early-stage HCC – *BCLC 0*). In early resectable HCC (*BCLC A*, encompassing either a single tumor or paucinodular disease <3 cm for each nodule, in patients with preserved liver function and good performance status), a meta-analysis comparing surgery versus RFA involving 574 patients did not reveal any significant differences in terms of mortality; however, recurrences were significantly more common after RFA [1]. A cost-effective analysis concluded that surgery for single large HCCs (3-5 cm) is the best treatment strategy [2]. RFA for paucinodular disease <3 cm remains an alternative option to surgical resection in appropriately selected candidates.

Microwave ablation (MWA) is a more effective treatment option for hepatocellular carcinoma (HCC), utilizing electromagnetic waves to generate heat and destroy cancer cells. It offers several advantages over other thermal ablation techniques, particularly in terms of speed, the size of the ablation zone, and reduced sensitivity to the heat-sink effect. Nonetheless, a phase II European randomized controlled trial (RCT) failed to identify any difference in efficacy compared to RFA for small HCCs [3]. A trend toward better performance of MWA has been observed in tumors larger than 3 cm, albeit at the cost of more complications.

A microwave antenna (probe) is inserted into the tumor under imaging guidance (ultrasound, CT). The microwave antenna emits electromagnetic waves that heat the surrounding tissue, creating a zone of thermal necrosis. This microwave energy (typically in the range of 900–2450 MHz) generates an oscillating electromagnetic field, which causes water molecules within the tumor tissue to oscillate, producing frictional heat. This heat raises the temperature of the tissue to levels (60–150°C) that cause coagulative necrosis of cancer cells. The size of this zone depends on the power and duration of the ablation.

In general, MWA can produce larger ablation zones than radiofrequency ablation (RFA), making it more effective for larger tumors. It also MWA heats tissue more rapidly, reducing procedure time. Most importantly, MWA is less affected by the heat-sink effect caused by nearby blood vessels, allowing for more consistent and effective ablation near vascular structures; therefore, MWA can achieve higher temperatures than RFA, potentially leading to more complete tumor destruction.

Cryoablation is an effective treatment for hepatocellular carcinoma (HCC), using extreme cold to destroy cancer cells. This technique has unique advantages, especially for tumors located in difficult-to-reach areas or near critical structures. Cryoablation involves the use of cryoprobes, which circulate a cryogen (usually liquid nitrogen or argon gas) to create extremely low temperatures, often as low as −160°C. The cryoprobes are inserted into the tumor under imaging guidance. The extreme cold leads to the rapid formation of ice crystals both inside and outside the cancer cells. Ice crystal formation causes mechanical disruption of cell membranes and intracellular structures, leading to cell death. Additionally, the freezing process disrupts blood flow to the tumor, causing further ischemic injury and cell death. After freezing, the tissue is allowed to thaw, which causes further cellular damage due to osmotic shifts and microvascular injury. This freeze-thaw cycle is often repeated to enhance tumor destruction.

An advantage of cryoablation is that the ablation zone can be precisely controlled and monitored using real-time imaging (ultrasound, CT), minimizing damage to surrounding healthy tissue. In addition, cryoablation is not affected by the heat-sink effect, making it suitable for tumors near large blood vessels. Monitoring can be easier with cryoablation, since the formation of the ice ball during the procedure is easily visible on imaging, allowing precise targeting and real-time monitoring. Lastly, patients often experience less post-procedural pain compared to heat-based ablation techniques.

Irreversible electroporation (IRE) is a relatively new, non-thermal ablation technique used for the treatment of hepatocellular carcinoma (HCC). IRE uses electrical pulses (typically in the range of 1500 to 3000 volts) delivered via needle electrodes placed in and around the tumor, to create permanent nanopores in cell membranes, leading to cell death while sparing the surrounding extracellular matrix and critical structures such as blood vessels and bile ducts. The disruption of the cell membrane homeostasis leads to irreversible cell injury and death. The process does not rely on heat, thereby minimizing thermal damage to the surrounding tissue. The extracellular matrix, including the collagen framework, remains intact. This preservation is crucial for maintaining the structural integrity of blood vessels, bile ducts, and other critical structures.

An important advantage of IRE is that it does not rely on thermal energy; thus, it avoids the complications associated with thermal ablation techniques, such as damage to blood vessels and bile ducts. The electrical fields can be precisely controlled, making it suitable for tumors located near vital structures. In addition, unlike thermal ablation methods, IRE is not affected by the heat-sink effect, making it effective for tumors adjacent to large blood vessels. Lastly, IRE can be safely repeated if necessary. However, there is a paucity of long-term data regarding the long-term efficacy of patients who undergo IRE for HCC.

3. Embolization techniques

In embolization procedures, a catheter is inserted into the branch(es) of the hepatic artery that supplies the tumor in the liver. Then, embolic agents, and occasionally chemotherapy, or both, are injected directly into the blood vessels to block or reduce the blood flow to the tumor. This deprives the tumor of oxygen and nutrients, leading to its shrinkage or destruction.

Transarterial embolization (TAE), or bland embolization, involves blocking the blood vessels feeding the tumor with embolic agents. Transarterial chemoembolization (TACE) combines the infusion of chemotherapy drugs with the embolization process. The choice between TACE and TAE depends on various factors, including the size and location of the tumor, liver function, and overall health of the patient.

Transarterial chemoembolization (TACE) is the predominant option for embolization techniques. It delivers chemotherapeutic regimens and embolization material to the arterial network, feeding the primary liver tumor. Following the publication of two landmark trials, TACE has been established as the first-line treatment for patients with intermediate-stage HCC (*BCLC B*) who suffer from unresectable liver-confined disease with no evidence of vascular invasion, preserved liver function, and good performance status [4, 5]. Conventional TACE (cTACE) uses a mixture of chemotherapeutic drugs and lipiodol, while drug-eluting beads TACE (DEB-TACE) uses embolic microspheres, which release the cytotoxic agents in a controlled manner. They are both equivalent in terms of survival, tumor response, and safety profile. Transarterial chemoembolization can also be offered in patients with earlier-stage HCC who are not candidates for surgical or ablative treatments. Furthermore, for patients on the waiting list to receive a liver transplant, TACE has successfully been used as a bridge to transplantation, reducing the drop-out rates.

Transarterial radioembolization (TARE), also known as *selective internal radiation therapy (SIRT)*, is another embolization option for HCC. TARE involves the delivery of radiation directly to the tumor in the liver using tiny radioactive particles called microspheres, such as Yttrium-90 (Y-90), which can emit high-energy radiation to the tumor. One of the main advantages is the fact that it can be used in patients with malignant portal vein thrombosis due to its minimal embolic effect. Yet, it carries the limitations of restricted availability and technically demanding procedures. It has been investigated in the setting of early, intermediate and advanced HCC. In early-intermediate-stage tumors, it has been suggested that TARE may lead to acceptable response rates or even serve as an effective downstaging strategy. Even though largely controversial, it may be an option in the context of multidisciplinary decisions for select patients. Future trials will explore the efficacy of intensive dosimetry TARE in this scenario. For advanced HCC, three RCTs have failed to provide any conclusive evidence of the survival advantage of TARE when compared to sorafenib; hence, TARE is not currently recommended in this setting [6–8].

3.1 Combination of ablative and embolization modalities

Combination of both techniques is feasible, albeit not universally incorporated in existing guidelines. TACE has the inert ability to reduce the "heat-sink" effect, which is the major drawback in the use of RFA, by embolizing the feeding arterial tumor vessels. It can also enhance the RFA-induced ablation zone and synergistically eradicate any micrometastatic satellite deposits. Sequential application of cTACE and RFA has been shown to improve the survival of patients with recurrent HCC lesions of less than 5 cm in diameter.

An important study from Winer et al. [9] evaluated all patients diagnosed with HCC (1998–2013) at New York University/Bellevue Hospital Center in New York City. Patients were retrospectively analyzed for date of diagnosis, treatment type, length of follow-up, and survival. Patients were excluded if they did not undergo TACE or RFA/MWA or underwent other treatments, such as surgery. The primary outcome was all-cause mortality 5 years after diagnosis. Of 509 patients diagnosed with HCC, 109 (21.4%) met inclusion criteria. Sixty were treated with TACE alone, 30 with ablation alone, and 19 were treated with both, either concomitantly or in sequence. Median follow-up and overall median survival were 15.5, 19, and 52 months for TACE, ablation, and dual therapy, respectively. Survival at 5 years was 11.9, 13.3, and 42.1% for TACE, ablation, and combination groups, respectively. Kaplan Meier analysis revealed a significant increase in survival in the combination therapy group vs. RFA or TACE alone at 5 years ($p = 0.0006$). However, there was no significant difference in survival when comparing TACE vs. RFA/MWA at 5 years ($HR = 1.18$, $p = 0.48$). The authors concluded that patients treated with combination embolization/ablation (TACE plus RFA/MWA) versus either modality alone benefited a longer survival.

A recently published long-term outcomes of a phase III RCT demonstrated that combinational treatment (TACE plus RFA) for patients with early-stage HCC achieved improved overall and recurrence-free survival over the RFA monotherapy, and the effect was specifically important for tumors larger than 3 cm [10].

3.2 Combination of locoregional therapies with systematic treatment

The concept relies on the fact that local thermal ablation or chemoembolization of primary liver tumors can change the tumor microenvironment and potentially reveal novel molecular targets, including the vascular endothelial growth factor receptor (VEGFR), the programmed death-1 cell surface receptor (PD-1) and its ligand (PD-L1). Local ablation can release various inflammatory cytokines and enhance the tumor's immunogenicity by sequestration of antigen-presenting cells and tumor-specific T-cells. On the other hand, transarterial chemoembolization induces, by definition, a local ischemic environment, which upregulates the expression of VEGFR, further promoting angiogenesis and local tumor recurrences. VEGF signaling *per se* has also been associated with immunomodulatory effects. Thereby, it has been suggested that the use of tyrosine kinase inhibitors (TKIs) or immune checkpoint inhibitors (ICIs) alone, in combination with each other, or with locoregional therapies, can provide significant benefits.

The phase III IMbrave 050 trial was the first to demonstrate positive results for adjuvant treatment in HCC [11]. It was reported that a combination of atezolizumab and bevacizumab significantly increased recurrence-free survival when compared to active surveillance in high-risk patients after resection or ablation with curative intent. Several other trials investigating the potential use of immunotherapy before or after local ablation are still ongoing.

As already mentioned, TACE is expected to exert a potentially synergistic effect in combination with TKIs by inhibiting angiogenesis and tumor proliferation. However, results from multiple RCTs have failed to confirm the expectations. TACTICS was the only trial to meet its primary endpoint for the treatment of intermediate HCC [12]. This RCT from Japan included 156 patients and compared the efficacy of cTACE plus sorafenib versus cTACE monotherapy. The median progression-free survival was 25.2 months in the combination treatment arm versus 13.5 months in the cTACE monotherapy arm (HR 0.59; 95% CI 0.41–0.87; $P = 0.006$). However, updated final outcomes of the same study failed to demonstrate a significant overall survival benefit. Lenvatinib is a multi-kinase inhibitor that has been approved as a first-line treatment option that is non-inferior to sorafenib in advanced HCC cases. An RCT recruiting 338 patients with advanced HCC reported significantly improved overall survival in patients receiving a combination of TACE with lenvatinib versus lenvatinib alone (median overall survival of 17.8 months versus 11.5 months; HR 0.45; $p < 0.001$) [13]. Alternative strategies, including the combination of PD-1/PDL-1 inhibitors with TACE are being investigated with increasing interest, and results are eagerly awaited.

Transarterial radioembolization combined with sorafenib was evaluated in the SORAMIC trial [8]. Yet, no overall survival benefit was observed. The potentially beneficial effects stemming from a combination of TARE with ICIs, even though initially encouraging, warrant further research.

4. Conclusion

The treatment of hepatocellular carcinoma (HCC), the most common type of primary liver cancer, depends on factors such as the stage and extent of the cancer, the patient's overall health and liver function, and the availability of resources and expertise. Treatment plans are often individualized based on a multidisciplinary

DOI: http://dx.doi.org/10.5772/intechopen.1005661

approach. Herein, we have presented the available options and have concluded that a combination of treatments is beneficial to the patient with HCC who is not a candidate for resection or transplantation.

Author details

Ioannis Margaris*, Nikolaos Arkadopoulos and Ioannis Hatzaras
Fourth Department of Surgery, Attikon University Hospital, National and Kapodistrial University of Athens, Athens, Greece

*Address all correspondence to: ihatzaras@gmail.com

References

[1] Majumdar A, Roccarina D, Thorburn D, Davidson BR, Tsochatzis E, Gurusamy KS. Management of people with early- or very early-stage hepatocellular carcinoma: An attempted network meta-analysis. Cochrane Database of Systematic Reviews. 2017;**3**(3):CD011650. Published 2017 Mar 28. DOI: 10.1002/14651858.CD011650.pub2

[2] Cucchetti A, Piscaglia F, Cescon M, et al. Cost-effectiveness of hepatic resection versus percutaneous radiofrequency ablation for early hepatocellular carcinoma. Journal of Hepatology. 2013;**59**(2):300-307. DOI: 10.1016/j.jhep.2013.04.009

[3] Vietti Violi N, Duran R, Guiu B, et al. Efficacy of microwave ablation versus radiofrequency ablation for the treatment of hepatocellular carcinoma in patients with chronic liver disease: A randomised controlled phase 2 trial. The Lancet Gastroenterology & Hepatology. 2018;**3**(5):317-325. DOI: 10.1016/S2468-1253(18)30029-3

[4] Llovet JM, Real MI, Montaña X, et al. Arterial embolisation or chemoembolisation versus symptomatic treatment in patients with unresectable hepatocellular carcinoma: A randomised controlled trial. Lancet. 2002;**359**(9319):1734-1739. DOI: 10.1016/S0140-6736(02)08649-X

[5] Lo CM, Ngan H, Tso WK, et al. Randomized controlled trial of transarterial lipiodol chemoembolization for unresectable hepatocellular carcinoma. Hepatology. 2002;**35**(5):1164-1171. DOI: 10.1053/jhep.2002.33156

[6] Vilgrain V, Pereira H, Assenat E, et al. Efficacy and safety of selective internal radiotherapy with yttrium-90 resin microspheres compared with sorafenib in locally advanced and inoperable hepatocellular carcinoma (SARAH): An open-label randomised controlled phase 3 trial. The Lancet Oncology. 2017;**18**(12):1624-1636. DOI: 10.1016/S1470-2045(17)30683-6

[7] Chow PKH, Gandhi M, Tan SB, et al. SIRveNIB: Selective internal radiation therapy versus Sorafenib in Asia-Pacific patients with hepatocellular carcinoma. Journal of Clinical Oncology. 2018;**36**(19):1913-1921. DOI: 10.1200/JCO.2017.76.0892

[8] Ricke J, Klümpen HJ, Amthauer H, et al. Impact of combined selective internal radiation therapy and sorafenib on survival in advanced hepatocellular carcinoma. Journal of Hepatology. 2019;**71**(6):1164-1174. DOI: 10.1016/j.jhep.2019.08.006

[9] Winer A, Rosen Y, Lu F, Berman RS, Melis M, Miller G, et al. Comparative effectiveness of combination TACE/ablation vs. monotherapy in hepatocellular carcinoma. Journal of Clinical Oncology. 2016;**34**(4_Suppl.):350

[10] Zhang YJ, Chen MS, Chen Y, Lau WY, Peng Z. Long-term outcomes of Transcatheter arterial chemoembolization combined with radiofrequency ablation as an initial treatment for early-stage hepatocellular carcinoma [published correction appears in JAMA Netw Open. 2022 Jan 4;5(1):e2148091]. JAMA Network Open. 2021;**4**(9):e2126992 [Accessed: Sep 1, 2021]. DOI: 10.1001/jamanetworkopen.2021.26992

[11] Hack SP, Spahn J, Chen M, et al. IMbrave 050: A phase III trial of

atezolizumab plus bevacizumab in high-risk hepatocellular carcinoma after curative resection or ablation [published correction appears in Future Oncol. 2020 Oct;16(29):2371]. Future Oncology. 2020;**16**(15):975-989. DOI: 10.2217/fon-2020-0162

[12] Kudo M, Ueshima K, Ikeda M, et al. Randomised, multicentre prospective trial of transarterial chemoembolisation (TACE) plus sorafenib as compared with TACE alone in patients with hepatocellular carcinoma: TACTICS trial. Gut. 2020;**69**(8):1492-1501. DOI: 10.1136/gutjnl-2019-318934

[13] Kudo M, Ueshima K, Saeki I, et al. A phase 2, prospective, Multicenter, single-arm trial of Transarterial chemoembolization therapy in combination strategy with Lenvatinib in patients with Unresectable intermediate-stage hepatocellular carcinoma: TACTICS-L trial. Liver Cancer. 2023;**13**(1):99-112. Published 2023 Jun 5. DOI: 10.1159/000531377

Chapter 5

Targeted Therapies for Hepatocellular Carcinoma Treatment

Dimitrios Dimitroulis, Christos Damaskos, Nikolaos Garmpis and Anna Garmpi

Abstract

Hepatocellular carcinoma (HCC) ranks among the most prevalent cancers globally, claiming the third spot in cancer-related fatalities. Surgery stands out as the optimal prognostic measure. Notable factors contributing to HCC encompass chronic viral infections, specifically hepatitis B virus (HBV) and hepatitis C virus (HCV), aflatoxins, tobacco use, and non-alcoholic fatty liver disease (NAFLD). The imperative task at hand is the creation of effective molecular markers and alternative therapeutic targets of substantial importance. This chapter delves into the overarching characteristics of HCC, offering insights into various targeted therapies that have propelled advancements in HCC treatment, underscoring the critical need for ongoing developments in this direction.

Keywords: cancer, carcinoma, hepatocarcinogenesis, hepatocellular, targeted, therapy

1. Introduction

Hepatocellular carcinoma (HCC) stands out as the predominant primary liver malignancy globally, presenting a significant health challenge, particularly in sub-Saharan African and Asian nations. It ranks as the fifth most common cancer diagnosis in males and the sixth in females, causing 250,000–1,000,000 deaths globally. The incidence of liver cancer exhibits considerable geographical variation. Extensive research has outlined the causative factors of HCC, including chronic hepatitis B virus (HBV), chronic hepatitis C virus (HCV), liver cirrhosis, non-alcoholic fatty liver disease (NAFLD), tobacco smoking, and consumption of aflatoxin rich foods. Notably, a higher incidence is observed in males due to the prevalence of chronic viral liver infections, tobacco smoking, and heavy alcohol consumption. Investigations are ongoing regarding the potential protective role of estrogens [1]. Orthotopic liver transplantation (OLT) is the favored treatment for terminal-stage patients, boasting 1-year survival rates of 80–90%. The imperative need for alternative treatment methods for terminal-stage patients is crucial, particularly in underdeveloped countries facing limited resources. Surveillance programs have been implemented in developed nations to identify high-risk HCC patients. However, resource constraints in underdeveloped regions often result in later-stage HCC presentations, precluding curative treatments [2]. Various imaging modalities are available for liver tumor evaluation, with Ultrasonography (US) emerging as a cost-effective screening method, surpassing computed tomography (CT) and magnetic resonance imaging (MRI) in terms of cost, absence of radiation exposure, and avoidance of contrast agent nephrotoxicity. US demonstrates 60% sensitivity and over 95% specificity for screening chronic liver disease (liver cirrhosis) and virus-infected patients [3]. When a liver nodule suggests HCC, further diagnostic investigation is necessary. Biopsy is recommended for confirmed HCC cases with nodules exceeding 2 cm and low serum alpha-fetoprotein (AFP), or when resection, ablation, or liver transplantation is not feasible. Importantly, biopsy is discouraged in cases of elevated AFP and suggestive imaging, with treatment following established guidelines [4]. The molecular and histopathological pathways of HCC initiation remain incompletely understood. Indications point to genetic changes in pre-neoplastic hepatic cells and the gradual accumulation of mutations as culprits in malignant transformation leading to HCC [5]. HCC can manifest as a single liver nodule or multiple nodules, categorized by pathologists into well, moderate, and poorly differentiated stages. Well-differentiated HCC closely resembles healthy hepatic cells, while poorly differentiated HCC exhibits distinct structures and characteristics compared to normal cells.

1.1 Liver lobule: The organization of hepatic parenchyma

The liver lobule, defined as the microscopic functional unit of hepatic parenchyma, comprises a central terminal hepatic venule surrounded by up to six terminal portal triads, forming a polygonal unit. Hepatocytes, arranged in a single-cell-thick layer between the central venule and terminal portal triad branches, produce bile. Blood flows from sinusoids on each side of hepatocytes to the central venule. Along the sinusoidal lining, diverse cells include hepatic stellate cells, lymphoid cells, and Kupffer cells—specialized macrophages with roles in phagocytosis and inflammatory response initiation. Liver stellate cells, rich in retinoid, contribute to liver fibrosis and cirrhosis in response to injuries [6].

Toxic substance exposure and immune responses in the liver induce inflammation through Kupffer and stellate cells, potentially leading to necrosis. Persistent inflammation may progress to liver fibrosis and cirrhosis, characterized by distorted anatomy, septa, nodule formation, and altered blood flow within liver lobules. Cirrhosis emerges as a prominent risk factor for HCC, with continuous liver cell necrosis and regeneration increasing exposure to mutagenic agents. This dynamic process results in genetic and epigenetic changes, transforming normal hepatic cells into dysplastic foci, liver nodules, and ultimately HCC [7].

1.2 Staging systems

In CT scans, HCC typically manifests as a focal nodule with early arterial phase enhancement and rapid contrast washout during the portal vein phase in a three-phase contrast study. Conversely, on MRI scans, HCC presents as a lesion with high signal intensity.

The prognosis of HCC hinges on both underlying liver disease and tumor characteristics, prompting the proposal of multiple staging systems. The TNM classification of malignant tumors (TNM) system, devised by the American Joint Committee of Cancer (AJCC), emphasizes tumor, lymph nodes, and metastasis. While TNM staging predicts disease prognosis post-tumor resection, it falls short in evaluating liver function. Notably, tumor characteristics remain predictive of the ultimate outcome [8].

The Barcelona clinic liver cancer (BCLC) staging system currently governs HCC management, aligning treatment options with patient outcomes. Stage 0 patients, with tumors smaller than 2 cm, normal portal pressure, and normal serum bilirubin, offer a favorable scenario for tumor resection, yielding long-term survival rates exceeding 75%. Patients with larger tumors, a single tumor smaller than 5 cm, or multiple tumors (none exceeding 3 cm) are candidates for liver transplantation or surgical excision based on cirrhosis status [9].

Contemporary HCC treatments, such as liver resection and orthotopic liver transplantation, serve as gold standard procedures. Diverse hepatectomy techniques, aided by ablation methods and transcatheter devices, contribute to hepatic surgery. Liver transplantation proves effective for HCC patients with tumors up to 5 cm or three lesions, each 3 cm or smaller, achieving a 5-year overall survival rate of 75% [5]. Due to the prevalent late-stage presentation of HCC, systemic and palliative therapies dominate treatment approaches. Notably, HCC displays resistance to chemotherapy, leading to a surge in the popularity of targeted therapies as a novel strategy against the disease [10].

1.3 Expression of growth factors

The vascularity of HCC is marked by structural and functional irregularities crucial for tumor development. Vascular secretion is imperative for HCC cell proliferation, with pro-angiogenic growth factors and their receptor tyrosine kinases (RTK) playing a significant role in angiogenesis within the tumor microenvironment [11]. Prominent growth factors such as vascular endothelial growth factor (VEGF), epidermal growth factor (EGF), fibroblast growth factor (FGF), insulin-like growth factor (IGF), and platelet-derived growth factor (PDGF) contribute to heightened vascularity and cancer cell proliferation, expressing not only in cancer cells but also in the surrounding healthy tissue. Their expression correlates with disease progression and vascular invasion [12].

RTKs are transmembrane proteins facilitating extracellular signal transduction that play a pivotal role in HCC development. Activated upon growth factor binding, RTKs initiate various intracellular signaling pathways, including PI3K/AKT/mTOR and RAS/RAF/MEK/ERK, fostering angiogenesis, cell survival, and the migration, proliferation, and differentiation of endothelial cells [13]. Dysregulation of RTKs, whether through genomic rearrangements, gain-of-function mutations, overexpression, or constant stimulation from overexpressed growth factors, results in sustained kinase activity [13, 14].

Rat sarcoma (RAS) and rapidly accelerated fibrosarcoma (RAF) participate in intracellular signaling cascades that activate gene expression [15]. RAS activation of RAF leads to mitogen-activated protein kinase kinase (MEK) activation, subsequently activating extracellular signal-regulated kinase (ERK) and regulating various intracellular substrates and gene expression associated with cell proliferation [16]. ERK activation is linked to cancer cell proliferation.

The expression of growth factors like EGF in tumors is linked to tumor invasion, while PDGF expression is implicated in metastasis. Endothelial cell proliferation significantly contributes to tumor infiltration into healthy parenchyma and vascular invasion [17].

The phosphatidylinositol-3 kinase (PI3K) pathway, pivotal for cancer cell proliferation and survival, is implicated in HCC. Activating AKT and subsequently phosphorylating mTOR, the PI3K pathway influences cell proliferation and survival. Suppression of apoptosis through BCL2 associated agonist of cell death (BAD) inactivation is also attributed to this pathway. Notably, phosphatase and tensin homolog (PTEN), a regulator of the PI3K pathway, undergoes downregulation in HCC cells, and its suppression is linked to tumor grade progression, tumor stage, and poor overall prognosis [18].

Tyrosine kinase-type receptors, including VEGF receptors (VEGFR), PDGF receptors (PDGFR), EGF receptors (EGFR), FGF receptors (FGFR), and IGF receptors (IGFR), play a crucial role in HCC development. Activation of these receptors initiates the intracellular RAS in the RAF/MEK/ERK pathway. AP-1 proteins such as c-JUN and c-FOS activate the expression of genes associated with cell proliferation and heightened vascularity [19]. The RAF/MEK/ERK pathway activation is implicated in HCC progression, particularly in HBV-related cases [20].

Among the investigated signaling pathways, the VEGF and VEGFR-mediated pathway is one of the most extensively studied. VEGF-A isoforms, particularly VEGF165, are overexpressed in various tumors and are associated with disease progression, invasion, metastasis, and poorer patient survival. Consequently, anti-angiogenic agents focusing on VEGF-A and VEGFR-2 are under development [21].

No dominant pathway has been identified, leading to the evaluation of drugs targeting individual pathways for HCC treatment. Due to HCC's high resistance to systematic chemotherapy, current efforts concentrate on identifying signal pathways and genes associated with carcinogenesis and chemotherapy resistance [22].

2. Results

2.1 Multi-targeted tyrosine kinase inhibitors: First-line treatment

2.1.1 Sorafenib

The pioneer in targeted therapy for advanced HCC is Sorafenib, approved by the American Food and Drug Administration (FDA). This oral molecular agent exerts simultaneous effects on multiple targets, inhibiting Raf-1 within the RAF/MEK/ERK pathway and RTK involved in angiogenesis and tumor progression [23].

The Sorafenib Hepatocellular Carcinoma Assessment Randomized Protocol (SHARP) trial, a pivotal phase III study, led to FDA approval. Involving 602 patients with advanced HCC, the trial demonstrated a marked advance in median overall survival (OS). More specifically, it went from 7.9 to 10.7 months (hazard ratio (HR) = 0.69, $p = 0.001$). Time to progression (TTP) radiologically also prolonged from 2.8 to 5.5 months (HR = 0.58, $p < 0.001$). While the overall response rate (ORR) was 2%, the Sorafenib group exhibited a significantly higher disease control rate (DCR) compared to the placebo group (43% vs. 32%, $p = 0.002$) [24].

Additional trials in Asia further validated the efficacy of Sorafenib, revealing increased OS (6.5 vs. 4.2 months, HR = 0.68, $p = 0.014$) and prolonged TTP (2.8 vs. 1.4 months, HR = 0.57, $p = 0.0005$). The partial response was 3.3%, and the DCR was notably higher in the Sorafenib group (53% vs. 12%, $p = 0.0019$) [25].

Subsequent analyses of SHARP trial data considered baseline patient characteristics, affirming that Sorafenib improved OS and DCR independently of these factors [26]. These findings solidified Sorafenib as the standard therapy for advanced HCC.

Sorafenib has also been investigated in combination therapies. In a phase II trial, Sorafenib followed by concurrent modified FOLFOX (folinic acid, fluorouracil, oxaliplatin) (mFOLFOX) exhibited promising efficacy against advanced HCC, albeit with moderate toxicity [27–29]. Another study explored the combination of Sorafenib with transarterial chemoembolization (TACE), demonstrating a favorable safety profile and high DCR [30]. Comparative studies, such as Sorafenib + TACE vs. TACE alone, consistently revealed superior outcomes with combination therapy [31].

However, a phase III trial assessing Sorafenib post-TACE failed to demonstrate a significant prolongation of TTP. No marked difference in OS was observed between the Sorafenib and placebo groups [32]. While Sorafenib shows promise in combination therapies, further studies are warranted to establish the optimal approach.

2.1.2 Lenvatinib

Lenvatinib, an oral multi-kinase inhibitor (MKI), hinders tumor cell proliferation and angiogenesis by targeting VEGFR1–3, FGFR1–4, PDGFR alpha, RET protein, and c-Kit protein. Following promising results in a phase II trial [33], the phase III REFLECT trial compared Lenvatinib to Sorafenib as a first-line treatment in 954 patients with advanced HCC. Lenvatinib demonstrated non-inferiority, with a median OS of 13.6 vs. 12.3 months for Sorafenib (HR = 0.92, 95% CI: 0.79–1.06), and a superior TTP of 8.9 vs. 3.7 months (HR = 0.63, 95% CI: 0.53–0.73, $p < 0.0001$). Lenvatinib also exhibited a higher response rate (24.1% vs. 9.2%, $p < 0.001$) [34].

Reanalysis of the REFLECT study suggested potential underestimation of Lenvatinib's favorable effect, primarily due to imbalances in AFP concentrations and additional treatments between the two groups [35].

2.1.3 Sunitinib

Sunitinib is a tyrosine kinase inhibitor (TKI), with anti-angiogenic and antitumor behaviors, that targets VEGFR-1–3, PDGFR (alpha and beta), c-KIT, FLT3, and RET. Initial phase II studies indicated antitumor activity but with notable toxicities [36–38]. Subsequent phase III trials comparing Sunitinib to Sorafenib as a first-line treatment demonstrated inferior OS with Sunitinib (7.9 vs. 10.2 months, HR = 1.30, $p = 0.0014$), leading to the premature closure of the study due to safety concerns [39].

Combination therapies, such as Sunitinib plus TACE, showed improved OS and TTP compared to TACE alone in certain studies [40, 41]. However, conflicting results emerged, indicating the need for further investigation to establish the efficacy and safety of such combinations [42].

2.1.4 Linifanib

Linifanib, an oral TKI targeting VEGFR and PDGFR, was compared to Sorafenib in a randomized phase III trial for first-line treatment. While Linifanib exhibited favorable outcomes in terms of TTP and ORR, it did not translate into improved OS compared to Sorafenib. Linifanib was also associated with a higher incidence of adverse events, leading to dose reductions/interruptions and discontinuations, suggesting lower tolerability than Sorafenib [43].

2.1.5 Erlotinib

Erlotinib is an orally administered inhibitor of EGFR tyrosine kinase [44]. EGFR has been identified as a factor contributing to the endurance of HCC cells against sorafenib. Inhibiting EGFR has shown augmented effectiveness of sorafenib, as demonstrated by Ezzoukhry et al., who utilized model cell lines (Huh7, Hep3B, HepG2) to assess the response of HCC cells to therapeutic agents. They observed a cooperative outcome of EGFR inhibitors and sorafenib on the activity of the RAF-MEK-ERK kinase cascade in HCC cells which are EGFR-positive [45].

The phase III SEARCH trial, a randomized, placebo-controlled, double-blind study, compared erlotinib and sorafenib with sorafenib as a monotherapy in patients with untreated, advanced HCC. With 720 participants meeting inclusion criteria, including unresectable HCC, Child-Pugh liver function class A, life expectancy greater than 12 weeks, and an Eastern Cooperative Oncology Group Performance Status (ECOG-PS) of 0 or 1, the trial did not detect a significant difference in the median OS between the two groups (9.5 vs. 8.5 months, HR = 0.929, p = 0.408). Additionally, no significant difference in TTP (3.2 vs. 4.0 months, HR = 1.135, p = 0.18) was observed. Thus, the addition of erlotinib to sorafenib did not improve survival in advanced HCC patients based on this data analysis [46].

Erlotinib has also been investigated in combination treatments. In a phase II trial evaluating the efficacy of gemcitabine, oxaliplatin, and erlotinib (G + O + E) in 26 HCC patients, a DCR of 42% at 24 weeks was achieved. The median progression-free survival (PFS) was 35 weeks, and the median OS was 26 weeks. The observed difference between PFS and OS was mainly attributed to cirrhosis-related deaths without disease progression [47].

2.1.6 Foretinib

Foretinib is an oral MKI targeting mesenchymal epithelial transition (MET), reactive oxygen species (ROS), recepteur d'origine nantais (RON), anexelekto (AXL), tunica interna endothelial cell kinase 2 (TIE-2), and VEGFR2. In a single-arm, phase I/II study conducted in Asia, foretinib's safety and efficacy were evaluated as a first-line treatment for advanced HCC in patients with Child-Pugh A liver disease. With a maximum tolerated dose of 30 mg/day showing no major toxicity, among 35 patients assessed for efficacy, foretinib exhibited a median TTP of 4.24 months (95% CI: 2.79–9.59). The DCR was 82.9% (95% CI: 66.4–93.4), and the median OS was 15.7 months [48].

Although foretinib shows efficiency against advanced HCC, the conclusive evidence is still pending, necessitating randomized phase III trials to confirm its efficacy.

2.1.7 Donafenib

Donafenib is a novel, oral, small-molecule MKI, a modified form of sorafenib with a trideuterated N-methyl group. Following promising results from phase I studies, a randomized, phase II/III trial was conducted in a China. The trial included 659 patients with advanced HCC and Child-Pugh A, who had not previously undergone systematic treatment. Among them, 328 were treated with donafenib, and 331 with sorafenib, with 594 having HBV-related HCC. Donafenib demonstrated a higher ORR and DCRs of 4.6% and 30.8%, respectively, compared to sorafenib (2.7% ORR and

28.7% DCR). Although the median PFS for donafenib vs. sorafenib was not significantly different (3.7 vs. 3.6 months, HR = 0.909; 95% CI: 0.763–1.082; p = 0.0570), a significant difference was observed in OS. Between donafenib and sorafenib the OS was 12.1 vs. 10.3 months (HR = 0.831; 95% CI: 0.699–0.988; p = 0.0245). Donafenib also demonstrated a more favorable safety profile, with significantly fewer drug-related grade ≥ 3 adverse events (AEs) and lower rates of dose interruptions and reductions than sorafenib [49].

Hence, donafenib could be considered as part of the first-line treatment for advanced HCC, particularly in selected populations.

2.2 Multi-targeted tyrosine kinase inhibitors: Second-line treatment

2.2.1 Regorafenib

Regorafenib is an oral MKI targeting VEGFR 1–3, TIE 2, PDGFR beta, FGFR, RET, KIT, RAF-1, and B-Raf. Initially approved for refractory colorectal cancer and gastrointestinal stromal tumors, regorafenib's efficacy and safety in HCC were evaluated in a phase II study, showing anticancer activity and acceptable tolerability. Subsequently, the RESORCE trial, a phase III, double-blinded, placebo-controlled study, assessed regorafenib in patients with disease progression after first-line sorafenib treatment. With 573 participants meeting inclusion criteria, regorafenib demonstrated improved median OS (10.6 vs. 7.8 months, HR = 0.63, $p < 0.0001$) and median PFS (3.1 vs. 1.5 months, HR = 0.46, $p < 0.0001$), along with significantly higher ORR (11% vs. 4%) [50].

The primary objective of this study was achieved successfully, suggesting that the sequential use of two MKIs with partly overlapping targets provides a survival benefit in HCC, especially for patients progressing after sorafenib treatment.

2.2.2 Cabozantinib

Cabozantinib is an oral TKI suppressing MET, VEGFR-2, and RET. A phase II randomized discontinuation trial (RDT) involving 41 HCC patients with Child-Pugh A liver function who had received 1 systemic agent or less, demonstrated a median OS of 11.5 months and a median PFS of 5.2 months [44]. Subsequently, the CALESTIAL trial assessed cabozantinib's efficacy in individuals with advanced HCC, specifically those with Child-Pugh A status and an ECOG-PS of 0 or 1, who had undergone one to two prior systematic treatments, including sorafenib. A total of 707 patients were randomly assigned to receive either 60 mg of cabozantinib once daily or a placebo. Following the second interim analysis, the trial achieved its primary goal, demonstrating a statistically significant and clinically relevant enhancement in median OS compared to the placebo group (10.2 vs. 8.0 months, HR = 0.76, 95% CI: 0.63–0.92, p = 0.0049). Secondary endpoints, including median PFS (5.2 vs. 1.9 months, HR = 0.44, $p < 0.001$) and ORR (4% vs. 0.4%, p = 0.0086), were also significantly improved [51]. In a post hoc analysis, patients who had previously received only sorafenib were included, revealing improved OS and PFS with cabozantinib regardless of the duration of prior sorafenib treatment [52].

Cabozantinib stands as a viable option for second- or third-line treatment in patients with advanced HCC.

2.2.3 Tivantinib

Tivantinib is a selective inhibitor of c-MET, a tyrosine kinase receptor encoded by the protooncogene c-MET. Upon attachment to hepatocyte growth factor (HGF), the MET signaling pathway is activated, influencing various cellular processes such as differentiation, angiogenesis, cell invasion, and metastasis. Dysregulated MET expression is implicated in several human cancers, including HCC, and is associated with a poorer prognosis [53].

Following phase I and Ib trials, a randomized phase II trial compared tivantinib to placebo as a second-line treatment in 71 patients. The analysis revealed a longer TTP in patients treated with tivantinib compared to placebo (1.6 vs. 1.4 months, HR = 0.64, 90% CI: 0.43–0.94, p = 0.04). Notably, in patients with high c-MET expression determined by immunohistochemistry, tivantinib demonstrated a more significant improvement in median TTP compared to placebo (2.7 vs. 1.4 months, HR = 0.43, 95% CI: 0.19–0.97, p = 0.03). Moreover, the median OS was better with tivantinib (7.2 vs. 3.8 months, HR = 0.38, 95% CI: 0.18–0.81, p = 0.01). However, the tivantinib group experienced higher and more severe cases of neutropenia and anemia, with four deaths attributed to neutropenia [54, 55].

Subsequently, a phase III study with 340 patients failed to demonstrate the effectiveness of tivantinib in unresectable HCC with radiographically confirmed progression after sorafenib-containing systemic therapy. No significant differences were observed in OS, PFS, TTP, or DCR between the tivantinib and placebo groups [56]. Another phase III study with 195 patients also did not show statistically significant results [57]. Thus, tivantinib has not been proven as an effective second-line agent, but the potential efficacy of concomitant inhibition of c-MET and VEGF warrants further investigation [56].

2.2.4 Axitinib

Axitinib is a highly effective inhibitor targeting VEGFR 1, 2, and 3 with specificity. In a phase II trial conducted without control group involvement, patients diagnosed with advanced HCC, ranging from Child-Pugh A to B7 status, and experiencing disease progression post-treatment with tyrosine kinase inhibitors (TKI)/antiangiogenic drugs were enrolled, the median OS for all patients was 7.1 months, and PFS was 3.6 months. The tumor control rate at 16 weeks was 42.3%, with one partial response and 10 stable disease cases. Adverse events led to treatment discontinuation in 26.7% of patients [58]. However, a randomized phase II study comparing axitinib to placebo in second-line treatment of advanced HCC did not demonstrate its superiority in terms of OS. The median OS was 12.7 months with axitinib/BSC and 9.7 months with placebo/BSC, but the difference was not statistically significant. Notably, excluding patients intolerant to prior antiangiogenic treatment showed a greater difference in OS, and PFS and TTP were significantly longer in the axitinib arm [59].

Axitinib's potential as a first-line treatment in combination with TACE also showed promising results in a phase II trial, with a 2-year survival rate of 43.7% and a median OS of 18.8 months [60]. In conclusion, axitinib exhibits significant antitumor activity in HCC, but further study through phase III clinical trials is crucial.

2.2.5 Anlotinib

Anlotinib is an orally administered TKI targeting VEGFR, FGFR, PDGFR, and c-kit. In a phase II clinical trial, two cohorts were studied for first-line and second-line treatments. Cohort 1, including 26 patients without prior TKI treatment, showed a 12-week PFS rate of 80.8% and a 24-week PFS rate of 54.2%. The median TTP was 5.9 months, and the median OS was 12.8 months. In cohort 2, including 24 patients with previous treatment, the 12-week PFS rate was 72.5%, with a 24-week PFS rate of 46.6%. The median TTP and OS were 4.6 months and 18.0 months, respectively. Anlotinib's safety profile was favorable, and patients with lower baseline plasma levels of CXCL1 showed longer TTP in both cohorts [61].

Anlotinib's efficacy was also explored in combination with penpulimab (Anti-PD-1) as a first-line therapy [62]. Overall, anlotinib demonstrates satisfactory efficacy in both first-line and second-line treatments for advanced HCC, emphasizing the need for further studies to confirm these findings and explore combination therapies.

2.2.6 Tepotinib

Tepotinib is an orally available, potent, and highly selective MET inhibitor. In a phase Ib study and subsequent phase II trial, tepotinib demonstrated positive outcomes in advanced HCC patients who had received at least 4 weeks of sorafenib treatment. The median TTP was 2.1 months, PFS was 1.5 months, and OS was 7.2 months. The DCR was 57.1%, with stable disease, complete response, and partial response observed. No major safety issues were reported, and patients with MET over-expression exhibited more favorable efficacy profiles [63].

In another phase Ib/II study with Asian patients, tepotinib improved TTP compared to sorafenib without significant toxicity. The median Independent Review Committee (IRC)-assessed TTP favored tepotinib, and the investigator-assessed TTP showed similar results. While there was no difference in OS, tepotinib demonstrated a higher DCR [64]. Tepotinib appears to be an efficient agent for both first- and second-line treatment in advanced HCC, particularly in patients with MET over-expression. Confirmatory evidence from phase III trials is necessary to validate these findings.

2.3 Anti-VEGF therapies

2.3.1 Ramucirumab

Ramucirumab is an injectable agent, a human IgG1 monoclonal antibody that selectively targets the extracellular domain of VEGFR2. By doing so, it obstructs ligand binding and hinders the stimulation of the receptor-mediated pathway in endothelial cells.

In a phase II trial, ramucirumab's potential as a first-line monotherapy for anti-cancer activity was investigated [65]. Subsequently, in the phase III REACH trial, its efficacy was evaluated as a second-line treatment in 565 patients with advanced HCC who had either failed treatment with sorafenib or were intolerant to it. Although no significant superiority in overall survival (OS) was observed (9.2 vs. 7.6 months, HR = 0.87, $p = 0.14$), secondary endpoints such as progression-free survival (PFS) (2.8 vs. 2.1 months, HR = 0.63, $p < 0.001$) and objective response (7% vs. <1%) favored the ramucirumab treatment arm. Further subgroup analysis was conducted, which identified efficacy in patients with an elevated baseline AFP level, particularly those with AFP ≥400 ng/mL (median OS 7.8 vs. 4.2 months, HR = 0.67, $p = 0.006$) [66].

Building on this observation, the REACH-2 study, a randomized phase III trial, focused on evaluating ramucirumab vs. placebo as second-line treatments in patients with AFP greater than 400 ng/mL. Enrolling 292 patients with BCLC stage B or C disease, refractory or not amenable to locoregional therapy, and Child-Pugh class A liver disease, the study demonstrated a statistically significant improvement in OS with ramucirumab (8.5 months; 95% CI: 7.0–10.6) compared to placebo (7.3 months [5.4–9.1]) with an HR = 0.710 (95% CI: 0.531–0.949), p = 0.0199. Additionally, PFS and DCR were significantly superior in the ramucirumab group [67].

Ramucirumab was also investigated in combination with emibetuzumab, showing potential anticancer activity in a phase Ib/II study across various solid tumors [19]. In summary, ramucirumab exhibits satisfactory efficacy in advanced HCC as a second-line treatment, particularly in a selected population with high AFP levels, and may hold promise in combination therapy.

2.3.2 Bevacizumab

Bevacizumab is a humanized monoclonal antibody that targets VEGF-A. Explored extensively for treating advanced HCC, several phase II trials have examined its safety and efficacy either as a monotherapy or in combination with other agents.

In a phase II trial with 46 patients, bevacizumab showed a median PFS of 6.9 months and a 1-year OS rate of 53%, reaching 28% and 23% at 2 and 3 years, respectively [68]. Another phase II trial with 38 patients reported a DCR of 42% at 16 weeks, a median PFS of 3 months, and a median OS of 8 months [69]. Notably, these studies enrolled patients with Child-Pugh A or compensated B, and observed adverse events were mainly hypertension and gastrointestinal bleeding.

Combination therapies involving bevacizumab, such as with gemcitabine and oxaliplatin or capecitabine and oxaliplatin, demonstrated potential anticancer activity in phase II studies [70]. Further exploration included combining bevacizumab with erlotinib, yielding promising results in some phase II studies, although others failed to show efficacy [71].

A randomized phase II study comparing bevacizumab plus erlotinib with sorafenib alone demonstrated comparable efficacy but better safety and tolerability for the combination [72].

Bevacizumab was also studied in combination with TACE. Although some trials showed potential efficacy, others revealed mixed results and safety concerns [73–75].

The pivotal shift in the treatment landscape occurred with a global, open-label, phase III trial comparing bevacizumab plus atezolizumab against sorafenib as a first-line treatment [76]. Atezolizumab, a programmed death 1 (PD-1) inhibitor, combined with bevacizumab, outperformed sorafenib, becoming the new standard of care. The trial demonstrated superior OS, PFS, and DCR with manageable safety issues [77]. Consequently, the combination of bevacizumab and atezolizumab is now considered the preferred first-line treatment for advanced HCC.

2.3.3 Apatinib

Apatinib stands out as a highly selective and potent TKI that effectively hampers angiogenesis by specifically targeting VEGFR2.

In a phase III trial, which was randomized, double-blind, placebo-controlled, and multicenter, the efficacy of apatinib as a second-line treatment for advanced HCC was evaluated. Among the 393 participants eligible for further analysis, 261 were assigned to the apatinib group, while 132 received a placebo. All participants had a Child-Pugh score of 7 or lower, with 41% having previously received sorafenib treatment. Approximately one-fifth of the participants had undergone more than one systematic therapy before receiving apatinib. The findings indicated a median overall survival (OS) of 8.7 months (95% CI: 7.5–9.8) in the apatinib group compared to 6.8 months (95% CI: 5.7–9.1) in the placebo group. The median progression-free survival (PFS) was 4.5 months (95% CI: 3.9–4.7) in the apatinib group and 1.9 months (95% CI: 1.9–2.0) in the placebo group, with a hazard ratio of 0.471 (95% CI: 0.369–0.601, $p < 0.0001$). The apatinib arm also exhibited higher rates of objective response and disease control. Adjusting for poststudy treatment further emphasized the efficacy of apatinib. Interestingly, the favorable effect appeared more pronounced in patients aged 65 years or younger, those with AFP ≥200 μg/L, those without previous sorafenib treatment, and those with only one previous systemic therapy. Notably, 12-month PFS and 12-month OS estimates showed overlapping 95% confidence intervals (CIs) between the apatinib and placebo groups. Treatment-related adverse events (AEs) were manageable, with hypertension being the most common grade 3 or 4 AE (28% of patients) [78].

Following encouraging results from a phase I study [79], a non-randomized, open-label, phase II trial explored apatinib's efficacy in combination with camrelizumab, a high-affinity, humanized IgG4-κ PD-1 monoclonal antibody. Enrolling 190 patients with advanced HCC and Child-Pugh A, the combination exhibited a promising ORR of 34.3% (first-line) and 22.5% (second-line). The 12-month survival rates were 74.7% and 68.2%, respectively. Median PFS for both cohorts demonstrated effectiveness at 5.7 months (first-line) and 5.5 months (second-line). Disease control rates were favorable, and safety profiles, though resulting in treatment discontinuation for 12.1% of patients, indicated a promising outcome [80]. A randomized, open-label, international, multicenter, phase III clinical study comparing this combination with sorafenib as a first-line treatment is currently underway (NCT03764293).

Furthermore, apatinib showcased positive outcomes in combination with TACE. In a single-center randomized controlled trial involving 44 patients with moderate and advanced HCCs and Child-Pugh A or B, the group receiving TACE plus apatinib demonstrated significantly prolonged Median PFS compared to the TACE-only group (12.5 vs. 6.0 months, $p < 0.05$). However, the reduction in AFP after 3 months and differences in ORR at 3, 6, 9, and 12 months were not statistically significant between the two groups [81].

In summary, apatinib has proven effective as a second-line treatment and shows promise in revolutionizing HCC treatment as part of combination therapies.

2.4 TGF-β receptor inhibitor

The TGF-β signaling pathway emerges as a therapeutic target for HCC. Galunisertib (LY2157299 monohydrate), an oral small-molecule inhibitor of TGF-β receptor I kinase, took center stage in a phase II trial evaluating its efficacy as a second-line treatment.

In this trial, 149 patients with advanced HCC and Child-Pugh class A or B7 were registered. Among them, 109 had AFP ≥1.5 × upper limit of normal (ULN) (Part A), and 40 had AFP <1.5 × ULN (Part B). The study revealed favorable results, with a median TTP of 2.7 months (95% CI: 1.5–2.9) in Part A and 4.2 months (95% CI: 1.7–5.5) in Part B. Median OS was 7.3 months (95% CI: 4.9–10.5) in Part A and 16.8 months (95% CI: 10.5–24.4) in Part B. The OS for Part A (150 mg twice daily) vs. Part B (150 mg twice daily) was significantly longer (HR = 2.1, 95% CI: 1.3–3.3). Responders to AFP demonstrated significantly longer TTP (4.3 vs. 1.5 months). The safety profile was notably favorable [82].

Exploring further, a phase II study assessed the combination of galunisertib and sorafenib as a first-line treatment in 47 patients. The study revealed a TTP of 4.1 months (95% CI: 2.8, 6.5) and OS of 18.8 months (95% CI: 14.8, 24.8). Prognostic value was observed for AFP and TGF-β1. Responders to TGF-β1 (decrease of >20% from baseline) exhibited longer OS (22.8 vs. 12.0 months, $p = 0.038$) [83].

In summary, therapeutic options for advanced HCC are provided by the TGF-β pathway, with galunisertib being extensively studied and showing favorable efficacy. However, further phase III trials are warranted to solidify these findings.

2.5 Immunotherapy

The immune system plays a crucial role in the body's defense against cancer, and immunotherapy has emerged as a promising strategy for cancer treatment. In the context of HCC, T-cells, a type of immune cell, are pivotal in recognizing and attacking tumor cells. T-cell activation is a complex process involving interactions with tumor-specific antigens and co-stimulatory signals. One key co-stimulatory signal involves the engagement of CD28 on T-cells with B7 molecules on antigen-presenting cells (APCs) [84]. However, this activation also triggers inhibitory pathways, such as the role of cytotoxic T-lymphocyte protein-4 (CTLA-4) and programmed cell death-1 (PD-1). CTLA-4, akin to CD28, binds to B7 molecules but suppresses T-cell responses. Similarly, PD-1, expressed by activated T-cells, B cells, and myeloid cells, interacts with its ligands PD-L1 and PD-L2 on APCs, leading to the downregulation of T-cell responses. Monoclonal antibodies (mAbs) targeting these immune checkpoints aim to enhance the anti-tumor immune response by inhibiting these inhibitory pathways, representing a novel and promising approach in cancer treatment [85].

2.5.1 Nivolumab

Nivolumab, a fully human immunoglobulin G4 monoclonal antibody targeting PD-1, has shown promise in treating advanced HCC. The CheckMate 040 trial assessed its safety and efficacy in patients with advanced HCC, including those with chronic viral hepatitis. The results demonstrated a response rate (RR) of 20%, DCR of 64%, and a median OS of 15 months. Notably, the manageable toxicity profile and positive responses led to FDA approval [86].

The combination of nivolumab and ipilimumab (anti-CTLA-4) was also evaluated in the same trial. Arm A, with nivolumab 1 mg/kg plus ipilimumab 3 mg/kg, showed an ORR of 32% and a median OS of 22.8 months, leading to FDA approval for second-line treatment of advanced HCC [87].

In the phase III trial (CheckMate 459), nivolumab was compared with sorafenib as a first-line treatment for advanced HCC. Nivolumab demonstrated a higher ORR (15%), a complete response rate of 4%, and a lower incidence of severe adverse events compared to sorafenib [88].

2.5.2 Pembrolizumab

Pembrolizumab, another anti-PD-1 monoclonal antibody, has shown efficacy in advanced HCC. In a phase II trial, pembrolizumab demonstrated an ORR of 17% and a DCR of 62% in patients previously treated with sorafenib [89]. A subsequent phase III trial (KEYNOTE-240) reinforced these findings, leading to FDA approval as a second-line treatment [90].

2.5.3 Avelumab

Avelumab, a fully human anti-PD-L1 monoclonal antibody, exhibited efficacy in advanced HCC in a phase II study. With a 10% ORR and a 73.3% DCR, avelumab demonstrated a median PFS of 3.5 months and a median OS of 14.2 months, making it a potential therapeutic option. Further research is needed to establish its role definitively [91].

2.5.4 Tremelimumab plus durvalumab

The combination of tremelimumab (anti-CTLA-4) and durvalumab (anti-PD-L1) has shown promise in a phase I/II study for second-line treatment of advanced HCC. The T300 + D arm exhibited the highest ORR (24%) and median OS (18.73 months). While effective, optimal dosage and potential monotherapy use require further investigation [92].

2.5.5 Sintilimab

Sintilimab, a selective anti-PD-1 antibody, in combination with IBI305 (bevacizumab biosimilar), demonstrated superiority over sorafenib in a phase II/III study (ORIENT-32) for first-line treatment of HBV-related advanced HCC. With a significant improvement in ORR, DCR, and OS, this combination presents a promising alternative for this specific patient population [93].

2.6 CAR-T cell therapy

Chimeric antigen receptor T-cell (CAR-T) therapy, established for hematological malignancies, is being investigated for its efficacy and safety in HCC. In a phase II trial targeting CD133, CAR-T cells demonstrated a manageable safety profile and encouraging clinical outcomes in patients with advanced HCC. Further studies are crucial to integrate CAR-T cell therapy into advanced HCC treatment strategies [94].

3. Discussion

Despite notable advancements and the wider array of therapeutic options available, the overall prognosis for HCC remains modest. The introduction of sorafenib marked a significant milestone, enhancing our comprehension of the disease and contributing to prolonged survival among patients. As the inaugural systematically approved TKI, sorafenib set the stage for progressing toward a curative approach. Subsequently, considerable headway has been achieved in this direction.

Although initial outcomes of various treatments fell short in comparison to sorafenib, the groundbreaking results from the IMBRAVE150 trial have revolutionized first-line advanced HCC treatment. This combination has now become the established standard of care, significantly improving OS for HCC patients [77]. The landscape of immunotherapy appears promising, offering reliable monotherapies or combination treatments in both first and second-line settings [77, 88, 90, 93]. Simultaneously, antiangiogenic therapies, including bevacizumab, ramucirumab, and apatinib, demonstrate substantial efficacy as second-line treatments [67, 78]. Combination therapies involving anti-PD-1 and anti-angiogenesis antibodies exhibit a more favorable anti-HCC efficacy by inhibiting tumor angiogenesis and curbing immunosuppressive cell activity in the tumor microenvironment. This fosters the re-expression of cytotoxic T cells, reinstating their antitumor effect [95]. The ongoing surge in clinical trials on antineoplastic agents, as evident from the 750-plus registered trials (https://clinicaltrials.gov [Accessed: November 13, 2022]), underscores the scientific community's keen interest in exploring novel therapeutic avenues.

Neoadjuvant therapy, exemplified by the promising results of dovitinib, an anti-angiogenesis factor, presents another potential avenue that warrants further exploration [96]. Concurrent application of TACE and systemic treatments demonstrates favorable outcomes [40–42, 75, 81].

In the realm of immunotherapy, there is much to unravel. While immunotherapy has showcased significant benefits in melanoma, its application in other cancers like pancreatic cancer and cholangiocarcinoma is noteworthy [97]. CAR-T therapy, particularly targeting Glypican-3 (GPC3) and anti-CD133, shows promise in HCC, backed by both in vitro and in vivo success and numerous ongoing clinical studies [97].

Exploring alternative pathways of carcinogenesis, such as the TGF-β-associated pathway, introduces additional treatment options [23]. Molecular enhancements to existing drugs, as seen with donafenib, a deuterated sorafenib derivative with improved safety, further diversify therapeutic choices [49]. Clinical studies investigating donafenib in combination with anti-PD1 agents are underway (NCT04612712, NCT04503902).

Addressing the challenge of second-line treatment post-intolerance or failure of the initial therapy is critical. While numerous agents show promise, especially in patients treated with alternatives like bevacizumab/atezolizumab or lenvatinib, the data on second-line agents necessitate thorough collection.

The evolving landscape of targeted therapies prompts a reevaluation of chemotherapy agents' efficacy in advanced HCC. Combinatorial treatments involving chemotherapy and targeted agents hold promise, although larger patient cohorts in phase III clinical trials are indispensable for conclusive results [27, 28].

Exploration of specific molecular targets, including long non-coding RNAs (lncRNAs) and micro-RNAs (miRNAs), remains largely pre-clinical. While several miRNAs and lncRNAs emerge as potential therapeutic targets, their clinical studies are limited, posing safety concerns [98]. The extensive use of mRNA vaccines during the COVID pandemic may expedite this research.

In the era of diverse therapeutic options, personalized treatment selection remains challenging. Ramucirumab's efficacy in patients with AFP ≥400 ng/mL is an established knowledge [66, 67]. Biomarkers like c-met expression for tivantinib and TGF-β1 for TGF-β receptor inhibitors could predict treatment responses [59, 60, 83]. Identification of five biomarkers related to OS and TTP after regorafenib treatment emphasizes the need for further studies to establish such connections [99].

The etiology of HCC plays a role in therapeutic response variability. Sorafenib may offer greater benefits in HCV-positive patients than in HBV-positive patients. Notably, donafenib, a modified sorafenib derivative, improves OS in HBV-related HCC, presenting a viable alternative [49]. Conversely, immunotherapy might not be as beneficial for NASH-related HCC, necessitating exploration of alternative strategies [100].

Most clinical trials involve patients with preserved hepatic function (Child-Pugh A or B7), leaving limited data for other patients. Cautionary use of sorafenib in patients with impaired hepatic function is suggested, while comprehensive studies on the safety of other treatment options in similar populations are imperative. Understanding the pathogenesis of HCC is crucial for improving OS, emphasizing the necessity for deeper insights into molecular complexities. The evolving era will likely rely on combination treatments, necessitating continued research into genomic alterations and the development of HCC stem cell lines for novel drug testing.

4. Conclusions

In summary, HCC stands as the predominant primary liver malignancy and a prevalent cancer type. Resistant to chemotherapy, HCC patients in terminal stages find orthotopic liver transplantation as the optimal treatment. Targeted therapies have emerged as a focal point in HCC treatment, with various drugs targeting different molecular pathways showing promise. Sorafenib, initially groundbreaking, was surpassed by the atezolizumab and bevacizumab combination. Many other drugs have demonstrated efficacy or are currently under evaluation. This comprehensive review not only outlines the mechanisms of action of these agents but also discusses their advantages and drawbacks. Notably, it compares the features of newly developed agents with established treatment regimes. Understanding the current knowledge on HCC management is crucial for guiding future studies, shedding light on potential perspectives, and facilitating the development of advanced drugs.

Author details

Dimitrios Dimitroulis[1*], Christos Damaskos[2], Nikolaos Garmpis[2,3] and Anna Garmpi[4]

1 Second Department of Propedeutic Surgery, Laiko General Hospital, Medical School, National and Kapodistrian University of Athens, Athens, Greece

2 Nikolaos Christeas Laboratory of Experimental Surgery and Surgical Research, Medical School, National and Kapodistrian University of Athens, Athens, Greece

3 Department of Surgery, Sotiria General Hospital, Athens, Greece

4 First Department of Propedeutic Internal Medicine, Laiko General Hospital, Medical School, National and Kapodistrian University of Athens, Athens, Greece

*Address all correspondence to: dimitroulisdimitrios@yahoo.com

References

[1] Dimitroulis D, Damaskos C, Valsami S, Davakis S, Garmpis N, Spartalis E, et al. From diagnosis to treatment of hepatocellular carcinoma: An epidemic problem for both developed and developing world. World Journal of Gastroenterology. 2017;**23**(29):5282-5294. DOI: 10.3748/wjg.v23.i29.5282

[2] Loho IM, Siregar L, Waspodo AS, Hasan I. Current practice of hepatocellular carcinoma surveillance. Acta Medica Indonesiana. 2018;**50**(4):353-360

[3] Tzartzeva K, Obi J, Rich NE, Parikh ND, Marrero JA, Yopp A, et al. Surveillance imaging and alpha fetoprotein for early detection of hepatocellular carcinoma in patients with cirrhosis: A Meta-analysis. Gastroenterology. 2018;**154**(6):1706-1718.e1. DOI: 10.1053/j.gastro.2018.01.064

[4] Benson AB, D'Angelica MI, Abbott DE, Abrams TA, Alberts SR, Anaya DA, et al. Guidelines insights: Hepatobiliary cancers, version 2.2019. Journal of the National Comprehensive Cancer Network. 2019;**17**(4):302-310. DOI: 10.6004/jnccn.2019.0019

[5] Chen J, Ma L, Peng N-F, Wang S-J, Li L-Q. A meta-analysis of the relationship between glutathione S-transferases gene polymorphism and hepatocellular carcinoma in Asian population. Molecular Biology Reports. 2012;**39**(12):10383-10393. DOI: 10.1007/s11033-012-1917-0

[6] Kietzmann T. Liver zonation in health and disease: Hypoxia and hypoxia-inducible transcription factors as concert masters. International Journal of Molecular Sciences. 2019;**20**(9):2347. DOI: 10.3390/ijms20092347

[7] Sakamoto M, Mori T, Masugi Y, Effendi K, Rie I, Du W. Candidate molecular markers for histological diagnosis of early hepatocellular carcinoma. Intervirology. 2008;**51**(Suppl. 1):42-45. DOI: 10.1159/000122603

[8] Kudo M. Diagnostic imaging of hepatocellular carcinoma: Recent progress. Oncology. 2011;**81**(Suppl. 1):73-85. DOI: 10.1159/000333265

[9] Forner A, Reig ME, de Lope CR, Bruix J. Current strategy for staging and treatment: The BCLC update and future prospects. Seminars in Liver Disease. 2010;**30**(1):61-74. DOI: 10.1055/s-0030-1247133

[10] Mokdad AA, Hester CA, Singal AG, Yopp AC. Management of hepatocellular in the United States. Chinese Clinical Oncology. 2017;**6**(2):21. DOI: 10.21037/cco.2017.04.04

[11] Shinkaruk S, Bayle M, Laïn G, Déléris G. Vascular endothelial cell growth factor (VEGF), an emerging target for cancer chemotherapy. Current Medicinal Chemistry. Anti-Cancer Agents. 2003;**3**(2):95-117. DOI: 10.2174/1568011033353452

[12] Moon WS, Rhyu KH, Kang MJ, Lee DG, Yu HC, Yeum JH, et al. Overexpression of VEGF and angiopoietin 2: A key to high vascularity of hepatocellular carcinoma? Modern Pathology. 2003;**16**(6):552-557. DOI: 10.1097/01.MP.0000071841.17900.69

[13] Madhusudan S, Ganesan TS. Tyrosine kinase inhibitors in cancer therapy. Clinical Biochemistry. 2004;**37**(7):618-635. DOI: 10.1016/j.clinbiochem.2004.05.006

[14] Kontomanolis EN, Koutras A, Syllaios A, Schizas D, Mastoraki A, Garmpis N, et al. Role of oncogenes and tumor-suppressor genes in carcinogenesis: A review. Anticancer Research. 2020;**40**(11):6009-6015. DOI: 10.21873/anticanres.14622

[15] Yip-Schneider MT, Klein PJ, Wentz SC, Zeni A, Menze A, Schmidt CM. Resistance to mitogen-activated protein kinase kinase (MEK) inhibitors correlates with up-regulation of the MEK/extracellular signal-regulated kinase pathway in hepatocellular carcinoma cells. The Journal of Pharmacology and Experimental Therapeutics. 2009;**329**(3):1063-1070. DOI: 10.1124/jpet.108.147306

[16] Kim SY, Park SG, Jung H, Chi S-W, Yu DY, Lee SC, et al. RKIP downregulation induces the HBx-mediated Raf-1 mitochondrial translocation. Journal of Microbiology and Biotechnology. 2011;**21**(5):525-528. DOI: 10.4014/jmb.1012.12023

[17] Zhao Z-C, Zheng S-S, Wan Y-L, Jia C-K, Xie H-Y. The molecular mechanism underlying angiogenesis in hepatocellular carcinoma: The imbalance activation of signaling pathways. Hepatobiliary & Pancreatic Diseases International. 2003;**2**(4):529-536

[18] Wu P, Hu Y-Z. PI3K/Akt/mTOR pathway inhibitors in cancer: A perspective on clinical progress. Current Medicinal Chemistry. 2010;**17**(35):4326-4341

[19] Harding JJ, Zhu AX, Bauer TM, Choueiri TK, Drilon A, Voss MH, et al. A phase Ib/II study of ramucirumab in combination with emibetuzumab in patients with advanced cancer. Clinical Cancer Research. 2019;**25**(17):5202-5211. DOI: 10.1158/1078-0432.CCR-18-4010

[20] Schmitz KJ, Wohlschlaeger J, Lang H, Sotiropoulos GC, Malago M, Steveling K, et al. Activation of the ERK and AKT signalling pathway predicts poor prognosis in hepatocellular carcinoma and ERK activation in cancer tissue is associated with hepatitis C virus infection. Journal of Hepatology. 2008;**48**(1):83-90. DOI: 10.1016/j.jhep.2007.08.018

[21] Ferrara N. Vascular endothelial growth factor and the regulation of angiogenesis. Recent Progress in Hormone Research. 2000;**55**:15-35. discussion 35-6

[22] Roberts LR, Gores GJ. Hepatocellular carcinoma: Molecular pathways and new therapeutic targets. Seminars in Liver Disease. 2005;**25**(2):212-225. DOI: 10.1055/s-2005-871200

[23] Antoniou EA, Koutsounas I, Damaskos C, Koutsounas S. Remission of psoriasis in a patient with hepatocellular carcinoma treated with sorafenib. In Vivo. 2016;**30**(5):677-680

[24] Llovet JM, Ricci S, Mazzaferro V, Hilgard P, Gane E, Blanc J-F, et al. Sorafenib in advanced hepatocellular carcinoma. The New England Journal of Medicine. 2008;**359**(4):378-390. DOI: 10.1056/NEJMoa0708857

[25] Cheng A-L, Kang Y-K, Chen Z, Tsao C-J, Qin S, Kim JS, et al. Efficacy and safety of sorafenib in patients in the Asia-Pacific region with advanced hepatocellular carcinoma: A phase III randomised, double-blind, placebo-controlled trial. The Lancet Oncology. 2009;**10**(1):25-34. DOI: 10.1016/S1470-2045(08)70285-7

[26] Bruix J, Raoul J-L, Sherman M, Mazzaferro V, Bolondi L, Craxi A, et al. Efficacy and safety of sorafenib in patients with advanced hepatocellular carcinoma: Subanalyses of a phase

III trial. Journal of Hepatology. 2012;**57**(4):821-829. DOI: 10.1016/j.jhep.2012.06.014

[27] Abou-Alfa GK, Johnson P, Knox JJ, Capanu M, Davidenko I, Lacava J, et al. Doxorubicin plus sorafenib vs doxorubicin alone in patients with advanced hepatocellular carcinoma: A randomized trial: A randomized trial. Journal of the American Medical Association. 2010;**304**(19):2154-2160. DOI: 10.1001/jama.2010.1672

[28] Goyal L, Zheng H, Abrams TA, Miksad R, Bullock AJ, Allen JN, et al. A phase II and biomarker study of sorafenib combined with modified FOLFOX in patients with advanced hepatocellular carcinoma. Clinical Cancer Research. 2019;**25**(1):80-89. DOI: 10.1158/1078-0432.CCR-18-0847

[29] Chao Y, Chung Y-H, Han G, Yoon J-H, Yang J, Wang J, et al. The combination of transcatheter arterial chemoembolization and sorafenib is well tolerated and effective in Asian patients with hepatocellular carcinoma: Final results of the START trial: Final analysis of START. International Journal of Cancer. 2015;**136**(6):1458-1467. DOI: 10.1002/ijc.29126

[30] Kotsifa E, Vergadis C, Vailas M, Machairas N, Kykalos S, Damaskos C, et al. Transarterial chemoembolization for hepatocellular carcinoma: Why, when, how? Journal of Personalized Medicine. 2022;**12**(3):436. DOI: 10.3390/jpm12030436

[31] Liu Q, Dai Y. Sorafenib combined with transarterial chemoembolization prolongs survival of patients with advanced hepatocellular carcinoma. Journal of BUON. 2020;**25**(2):945-951

[32] Kudo M, Imanaka K, Chida N, Nakachi K, Tak W-Y, Takayama T, et al. Phase III study of sorafenib after transarterial chemoembolisation in Japanese and Korean patients with unresectable hepatocellular carcinoma. European Journal of Cancer. 2011;**47**(14):2117-2127. DOI: 10.1016/j.ejca.2011.05.007

[33] Ikeda K, Kudo M, Kawazoe S, Osaki Y, Ikeda M, Okusaka T, et al. Phase 2 study of lenvatinib in patients with advanced hepatocellular carcinoma. Journal of Gastroenterology. 2017;**52**(4):512-519. DOI: 10.1007/s00535-016-1263-4

[34] Kudo M, Finn RS, Qin S, Han K-H, Ikeda K, Piscaglia F, et al. Lenvatinib versus sorafenib in first-line treatment of patients with unresectable hepatocellular carcinoma: A randomised phase 3 non-inferiority trial. Lancet. 2018;**391**(10126):1163-1173. DOI: 10.1016/S0140-6736(18)30207-1

[35] Briggs A, Daniele B, Dick K, Evans TRJ, Galle PR, Hubner RA, et al. Covariate-adjusted analysis of the Phase 3 REFLECT study of lenvatinib versus sorafenib in the treatment of unresectable hepatocellular carcinoma. British Journal of Cancer. 2020;**122**(12):1754-1759. DOI: 10.1038/s41416-020-0817-7

[36] Faivre S, Raymond E, Boucher E, Douillard J, Lim HY, Kim JS, et al. Safety and efficacy of sunitinib in patients with advanced hepatocellular carcinoma: An open-label, multicentre, phase II study. The Lancet Oncology. 2009;**10**(8):794-800. DOI: 10.1016/S1470-2045(09)70171-8

[37] Zhu AX, Sahani DV, Duda DG, di Tomaso E, Ancukiewicz M, Catalano OA, et al. Efficacy, safety, and potential biomarkers of sunitinib monotherapy in advanced hepatocellular carcinoma: A phase II study. Journal of

Clinical Oncology. 2009;**27**(18):3027-3035. DOI: 10.1200/JCO.2008.20.9908

[38] Koeberle D, Montemurro M, Samaras P, Majno P, Simcock M, Limacher A, et al. Continuous Sunitinib treatment in patients with advanced hepatocellular carcinoma: A Swiss Group for Clinical Cancer Research (SAKK) and Swiss Association for the Study of the Liver (SASL) multicenter phase II trial (SAKK 77/06). The Oncologist. 2010;**15**(3):285-292. DOI: 10.1634/theoncologist.2009-0316

[39] Cheng A-L, Kang Y-K, Lin D-Y, Park J-W, Kudo M, Qin S, et al. Sunitinib versus sorafenib in advanced hepatocellular cancer: Results of a randomized phase III trial. Journal of Clinical Oncology. 2013;**31**(32):4067-4075. DOI: 10.1200/JCO.2012.45.8372

[40] Chen J, Zhou C, Long Y, Yin X. Sunitinib combined with transarterial chemoembolization versus transarterial chemoembolization alone for advanced-stage hepatocellular carcinoma: A propensity score matching study. Tumour Biology. 2015;**36**(1):183-191. DOI: 10.1007/s13277-014-2608-3

[41] Pokuri VK, Tomaszewski GM, Ait-Oudhia S, Groman A, Khushalani NI, Lugade AA, et al. Efficacy, safety, and potential biomarkers of sunitinib and transarterial chemoembolization (TACE) combination in advanced hepatocellular carcinoma (HCC): Phase II trial. American Journal of Clinical Oncology. 2018;**41**(4):332-338. DOI: 10.1097/COC.0000000000000286

[42] Xu Q, Huang Y, Shi H, Song Q, Xu Y. Sunitinib versus sorafenib plus transarterial chemoembolization for inoperable hepatocellular carcinoma patients. Journal of BUON. 2018;**23**(1):193-199

[43] Grothey A, Van Cutsem E, Sobrero A, Siena S, Falcone A, Ychou M, et al. Regorafenib monotherapy for previously treated metastatic colorectal cancer (CORRECT): An international, multicentre, randomised, placebo-controlled, phase 3 trial. Lancet. 2013;**381**(9863):303-312. DOI: 10.1016/S0140-6736(12)61900-X

[44] Kelley RK, Verslype C, Cohn AL, Yang T-S, Su W-C, Burris H, et al. Cabozantinib in hepatocellular carcinoma: Results of a phase 2 placebo-controlled randomized discontinuation study. Annals of Oncology. 2017;**28**(3):528-534. DOI: 10.1093/annonc/mdw651

[45] Ezzoukhry Z, Louandre C, Trécherel E, Godin C, Chauffert B, Dupont S, et al. EGFR activation is a potential determinant of primary resistance of hepatocellular carcinoma cells to sorafenib. International Journal of Cancer. 2012;**131**(12):2961-2969. DOI: 10.1002/ijc.27604

[46] Zhu AX, Rosmorduc O, Evans TRJ, Ross PJ, Santoro A, Carrilho FJ, et al. SEARCH: A phase III, randomized, double-blind, placebo-controlled trial of sorafenib plus erlotinib in patients with advanced hepatocellular carcinoma. Journal of Clinical Oncology. 2015;**33**(6):559-566. DOI: 10.1200/JCO.2013.53.7746

[47] Patt YZ, Murad W, Fekrazad MH, Baron AD, Bansal P, Boumber Y, et al. INST OX-05-024: First line gemcitabine, oxaliplatin, and erlotinib for primary hepatocellular carcinoma and bile duct cancers: A multicenter Phase II trial. Cancer Medicine. 2017;**6**(9):2042-2051. DOI: 10.1002/cam4.1138

[48] Yau TCC, Lencioni R, Sukeepaisarnjaroen W, Chao Y, Yen C-J, Lausoontornsiri W, et al.

A phase I/II multicenter study of single-agent foretinib as first-line therapy in patients with advanced hepatocellular carcinoma. Clinical Cancer Research. 2017;**23**(10):2405-2413. DOI: 10.1158/1078-0432.CCR-16-1789

[49] Qin S, Bi F, Gu S, Bai Y, Chen Z, Wang Z, et al. Donafenib versus sorafenib in first-line treatment of unresectable or metastatic hepatocellular carcinoma: A randomized, open-label, parallel-controlled phase II-III trial. Journal of Clinical Oncology. 2021;**39**(27):3002-3011. DOI: 10.1200/JCO.21.00163

[50] Bruix J, Tak W-Y, Gasbarrini A, Santoro A, Colombo M, Lim H-Y, et al. Regorafenib as second-line therapy for intermediate or advanced hepatocellular carcinoma: Multicentre, open-label, phase II safety study. European Journal of Cancer. 2013;**49**(16):3412-3419. DOI: 10.1016/j.ejca.2013.05.028

[51] Abou-Alfa GK, Meyer T, Cheng A-L, El-Khoueiry AB, Rimassa L, Ryoo B-Y, et al. Cabozantinib (C) versus placebo (P) in patients (pts) with advanced hepatocellular carcinoma (HCC) who have received prior sorafenib: Results from the randomized phase III CELESTIAL trial. Journal of Clinical Oncology. 2018;**36**(4_suppl):207. DOI: 10.1200/jco.2018.36.4_suppl.207

[52] Kelley RK, Ryoo B-Y, Merle P, Park J-W, Bolondi L, Chan SL, et al. Second-line cabozantinib after sorafenib treatment for advanced hepatocellular carcinoma: A subgroup analysis of the phase 3 CELESTIAL trial. ESMO Open. 2020;**5**(4):e000714. DOI: 10.1136/esmoopen-2020-000714

[53] Goldman JW, Laux I, Chai F, Savage RE, Ferrari D, Garmey EG, et al. Phase 1 dose-escalation trial evaluating the combination of the selective MET (mesenchymal-epithelial transition factor) inhibitor tivantinib (ARQ 197) plus erlotinib. Cancer. 2012;**118**(23):5903-5911. DOI: 10.1002/cncr.27575

[54] Santoro A, Rimassa L, Borbath I, Daniele B, Salvagni S, Van Laethem JL, et al. Tivantinib for second-line treatment of advanced hepatocellular carcinoma: A randomised, placebo-controlled phase 2 study. The Lancet Oncology. 2013;**14**(1):55-63. DOI: 10.1016/S1470-2045(12)70490-4

[55] Rimassa L, Santoro A, Daniele B, Germano D, Gasbarrini A, Salvagni S, et al. Tivantinib, a new option for second-line treatment of advanced hepatocellular carcinoma? The experience of Italian centers. Tumori. 2015;**101**(2):139-143. DOI: 10.5301/tj.5000217

[56] Rimassa L, Assenat E, Peck-Radosavljevic M, Pracht M, Zagonel V, Mathurin P, et al. Tivantinib for second-line treatment of MET-high, advanced hepatocellular carcinoma (METIV-HCC): A final analysis of a phase 3, randomised, placebo-controlled study. The Lancet Oncology. 2018;**19**(5):682-693. DOI: 10.1016/S1470-2045(18)30146-3

[57] Kudo M, Morimoto M, Moriguchi M, Izumi N, Takayama T, Yoshiji H, et al. A randomized, double-blind, placebo-controlled, phase 3 study of tivantinib in Japanese patients with MET-high hepatocellular carcinoma. Cancer Science. 2020;**111**(10):3759-3769. DOI: 10.1111/cas.14582

[58] McNamara MG, Le LW, Horgan AM, Aspinall A, Burak KW, Dhani N, et al. A phase II trial of second-line axitinib following prior antiangiogenic therapy in advanced hepatocellular carcinoma: Axitinib as Second-Line Treatment in HCC. Cancer. 2015;**121**(10):1620-1627. DOI: 10.1002/cncr.29227

[59] Kang Y-K, Yau T, Park J-W, Lim HY, Lee T-Y, Obi S, et al. Randomized phase II study of axitinib versus placebo plus best supportive care in second-line treatment of advanced hepatocellular carcinoma. Annals of Oncology. 2015;**26**(12):2457-2463. DOI: 10.1093/annonc/mdv388

[60] Chan SL, Yeo W, Mo F, Chan AWH, Koh J, Li L, et al. A phase 2 study of the efficacy and biomarker on the combination of transarterial chemoembolization and axitinib in the treatment of inoperable hepatocellular carcinoma. Cancer. 2017;**123**(20):3977-3985. DOI: 10.1002/cncr.30825

[61] Sun Y, Zhou A, Zhang W, Jiang Z, Chen B, Zhao J, et al. Anlotinib in the treatment of advanced hepatocellular carcinoma: An open-label phase II study (ALTER-0802 study). Hepatology International. 2021;**15**(3):621-629. DOI: 10.1007/s12072-021-10171-0

[62] Han C, Ye S, Hu C, Shen L, Qin Q, Bai Y, et al. Clinical activity and safety of penpulimab (anti-PD-1) with anlotinib as first-line therapy for unresectable hepatocellular carcinoma: An open-label, multicenter, phase Ib/II trial (AK105-203). Frontiers in Oncology. 2021;**11**:684867. DOI: 10.3389/fonc.2021.684867

[63] Decaens T, Barone C, Assenat E, Wermke M, Fasolo A, Merle P, et al. Phase 1b/2 trial of tepotinib in sorafenib pretreated advanced hepatocellular carcinoma with MET overexpression. British Journal of Cancer. 2021;**125**(2):190-199. DOI: 10.1038/s41416-021-01334-9

[64] Ryoo B-Y, Cheng A-L, Ren Z, Kim T-Y, Pan H, Rau K-M, et al. Randomised Phase 1b/2 trial of tepotinib vs sorafenib in Asian patients with advanced hepatocellular carcinoma with MET overexpression. British Journal of Cancer. 2021;**125**(2):200-208. DOI: 10.1038/s41416-021-01380-3

[65] Zhu AX, Finn RS, Mulcahy M, Gurtler J, Sun W, Schwartz JD, et al. A phase II and biomarker study of ramucirumab, a human monoclonal antibody targeting the VEGF receptor-2, as first-line monotherapy in patients with advanced hepatocellular cancer. Clinical Cancer Research. 2013;**19**(23):6614-6623. DOI: 10.1158/1078-0432.CCR-13-1442

[66] Zhu AX, Park JO, Ryoo B-Y, Yen C-J, Poon R, Pastorelli D, et al. Ramucirumab versus placebo as second-line treatment in patients with advanced hepatocellular carcinoma following first-line therapy with sorafenib (REACH): A randomised, double-blind, multicentre, phase 3 trial. The Lancet Oncology. 2015;**16**(7):859-870. DOI: 10.1016/S1470-2045(15)00050-9

[67] Zhu AX, Kang Y-K, Yen C-J, Finn RS, Galle PR, Llovet JM, et al. Ramucirumab after sorafenib in patients with advanced hepatocellular carcinoma and increased α-fetoprotein concentrations (REACH-2): A randomised, double-blind, placebo-controlled, phase 3 trial. The Lancet Oncology. 2019;**20**(2):282-296. DOI: 10.1016/S1470-2045(18)30937-9

[68] Siegel AB, Cohen EI, Ocean A, Lehrer D, Goldenberg A, Knox JJ, et al. Phase II trial evaluating the clinical and biologic effects of bevacizumab in unresectable hepatocellular carcinoma. Journal of Clinical Oncology. 2008;**26**(18):2992-2998. DOI: 10.1200/JCO.2007.15.9947

[69] Boige V, Malka D, Bourredjem A, Dromain C, Baey C, Jacques N, et al. Efficacy, safety, and biomarkers of single-agent bevacizumab therapy in patients with advanced hepatocellular carcinoma. The Oncologist.

2012;**17**(8):1063-1072. DOI: 10.1634/theoncologist.2011-0465

[70] Sun W, Sohal D, Haller DG, Mykulowycz K, Rosen M, Soulen MC, et al. Phase 2 trial of bevacizumab, capecitabine, and oxaliplatin in treatment of advanced hepatocellular carcinoma. Cancer. 2011;**117**(14):3187-3192. DOI: 10.1002/cncr.25889

[71] Philip PA, Mahoney MR, Holen KD, Northfelt DW, Pitot HC, Picus J, et al. Phase 2 study of bevacizumab plus erlotinib in patients with advanced hepatocellular cancer. Cancer. 2012;**118**(9):2424-2430. DOI: 10.1002/cncr.26556

[72] Thomas MB, Garrett-Mayer E, Anis M, Anderton K, Bentz T, Edwards A, et al. A randomized phase II open-label multi-institution study of the combination of bevacizumab and erlotinib compared to sorafenib in the first-line treatment of patients with advanced hepatocellular carcinoma. Oncology. 2018;**94**(6):329-339. DOI: 10.1159/000485384

[73] Buijs M, Reyes DK, Pawlik TM, Blackford AL, Salem R, Messersmith WA, et al. Phase 2 trial of concurrent bevacizumab and transhepatic arterial chemoembolization in patients with unresectable hepatocellular carcinoma. Cancer. 2013;**119**(5):1042-1049. DOI: 10.1002/cncr.27859

[74] Britten CD, Gomes AS, Wainberg ZA, Elashoff D, Amado R, Xin Y, et al. Transarterial chemoembolization plus or minus intravenous bevacizumab in the treatment of hepatocellular cancer: A pilot study. BMC Cancer. 2012;**12**(1):16. DOI: 10.1186/1471-2407-12-16

[75] Pinter M, Ulbrich G, Sieghart W, Kölblinger C, Reiberger T, Li S, et al. Hepatocellular carcinoma: A phase II randomized controlled double-blind trial of transarterial chemoembolization in combination with biweekly intravenous administration of bevacizumab or a placebo. Radiology. 2015;**277**(3):903-912. DOI: 10.1148/radiol.2015142140

[76] Lee MS, Ryoo B-Y, Hsu C-H, Numata K, Stein S, Verret W, et al. Atezolizumab with or without bevacizumab in unresectable hepatocellular carcinoma (GO30140): An open-label, multicentre, phase 1b study. The Lancet Oncology. 2020;**21**(6):808-820. DOI: 10.1016/s1470-2045(20)30156-x

[77] Finn RS, Qin S, Ikeda M, Galle PR, Ducreux M, Kim T-Y, et al. Atezolizumab plus bevacizumab in unresectable hepatocellular carcinoma. The New England Journal of Medicine. 2020;**382**(20):1894-1905. DOI: 10.1056/NEJMoa1915745

[78] Qin S, Li Q, Gu S, Chen X, Lin L, Wang Z, et al. Apatinib as second-line or later therapy in patients with advanced hepatocellular carcinoma (AHELP): A multicentre, double-blind, randomised, placebo-controlled, phase 3 trial. The Lancet Gastroenterology & Hepatology. 2021;**6**(7):559-568. DOI: 10.1016/s2468-1253(21)00109-6

[79] Xu J, Zhang Y, Jia R, Yue C, Chang L, Liu R, et al. Anti-PD-1 antibody SHR-1210 combined with apatinib for advanced hepatocellular carcinoma, gastric, or esophagogastric junction cancer: An open-label, dose escalation and expansion study. Clinical Cancer Research. 2019;**25**(2):515-523. DOI: 10.1158/1078-0432.ccr-18-2484

[80] Xu J, Shen J, Gu S, Zhang Y, Wu L, Wu J, et al. Camrelizumab in combination with apatinib in patients with advanced hepatocellular carcinoma

(RESCUE): A nonrandomized, open-label, phase II trial. Clinical Cancer Research. 2021;**27**(4):1003-1011. DOI: 10.1158/1078-0432.CCR-20-2571

[81] Lu W, Jin X-L, Yang C, Du P, Jiang F-Q, Ma J-P, et al. Comparison of efficacy between TACE combined with apatinib and TACE alone in the treatment of intermediate and advanced hepatocellular carcinoma: A single-center randomized controlled trial. Cancer Biology & Therapy. 2017;**18**(6):433-438. DOI: 10.1080/15384047.2017.1323589

[82] Faivre S, Santoro A, Kelley RK, Gane E, Costentin CE, Gueorguieva I, et al. Novel transforming growth factor beta receptor I kinase inhibitor galunisertib (LY2157299) in advanced hepatocellular carcinoma. Liver International. 2019;**39**(8):1468-1477. DOI: 10.1111/liv.14113

[83] Kelley RK, Gane E, Assenat E, Siebler J, Galle PR, Merle P, et al. A phase 2 study of galunisertib (TGF-β1 receptor type I inhibitor) and sorafenib in patients with advanced hepatocellular carcinoma. Clinical and Translational Gastroenterology. 2019;**10**(7):e00056. DOI: 10.14309/ctg.0000000000000056

[84] Linsley PS. Distinct roles for CD28 and cytotoxic T lymphocyte-associated molecule-4 receptors during T cell activation? The Journal of Experimental Medicine. 1995;**182**(2):289-292. DOI: 10.1084/jem.182.2.289

[85] Ilyas FZ, Beane JD, Pawlik TM. The state of immunotherapy in hepatobiliary cancers. Cells. 2021;**10**(8):2096. DOI: 10.3390/cells10082096

[86] El-Khoueiry AB, Sangro B, Yau T, Crocenzi TS, Kudo M, Hsu C, et al. Nivolumab in patients with advanced hepatocellular carcinoma (CheckMate 040): An open-label, non-comparative, phase 1/2 dose escalation and expansion trial. Lancet. 2017;**389**(10088):2492-2502. DOI: 10.1016/S0140-6736(17)31046-2

[87] Yau T, Kang Y-K, Kim T-Y, El-Khoueiry AB, Santoro A, Sangro B, et al. Efficacy and safety of nivolumab plus ipilimumab in patients with advanced hepatocellular carcinoma previously treated with sorafenib: The CheckMate 040 randomized clinical trial. JAMA Oncology. 2020;**6**(11):e204564. DOI: 10.1001/jamaoncol.2020.4564

[88] Yau T, Park J-W, Finn RS, Cheng A-L, Mathurin P, Edeline J, et al. Nivolumab versus sorafenib in advanced hepatocellular carcinoma (CheckMate 459): A randomised, multicentre, open-label, phase 3 trial. The Lancet Oncology. 2022;**23**(1):77-90. DOI: 10.1016/s1470-2045(21)00604-5

[89] Zhu AX, Finn RS, Edeline J, Cattan S, Ogasawara S, Palmer D, et al. Pembrolizumab in patients with advanced hepatocellular carcinoma previously treated with sorafenib (KEYNOTE-224): A non-randomised, open-label phase 2 trial. The Lancet Oncology. 2018;**19**(7):940-952. DOI: 10.1016/s1470-2045(18)30351-6

[90] Finn RS, Ryoo B-Y, Merle P, Kudo M, Bouattour M, Lim HY, et al. Pembrolizumab as second-line therapy in patients with advanced hepatocellular carcinoma in KEYNOTE-240: A randomized, double-blind, phase III trial. Journal of Clinical Oncology. 2020;**38**(3):193-202. DOI: 10.1200/JCO.19.01307

[91] Lee D-W, Cho EJ, Lee J-H, Yu SJ, Kim YJ, Yoon J-H, et al. Phase II study of avelumab in patients with advanced hepatocellular carcinoma previously

treated with sorafenib. Clinical Cancer Research. 2021;**27**(3):713-718. DOI: 10.1158/1078-0432.CCR-20-3094

[92] Kelley RK, Sangro B, Harris W, Ikeda M, Okusaka T, Kang Y-K, et al. Safety, efficacy, and pharmacodynamics of tremelimumab plus durvalumab for patients with unresectable hepatocellular carcinoma: Randomized expansion of a phase I/II study. Journal of Clinical Oncology. 2021;**39**(27):2991-3001. DOI: 10.1200/jco.20.03555

[93] Ren Z, Xu J, Bai Y, Xu A, Cang S, Du C, et al. Sintilimab plus a bevacizumab biosimilar (IBI305) versus sorafenib in unresectable hepatocellular carcinoma (ORIENT-32): A randomised, open-label, phase 2-3 study. The Lancet Oncology. 2021;**22**(7):977-990. DOI: 10.1016/s1470-2045(21)00252-7

[94] Dai H, Tong C, Shi D, Chen M, Guo Y, Chen D, et al. Efficacy and biomarker analysis of CD133-directed CAR T cells in advanced hepatocellular carcinoma: A single-arm, open-label, phase II trial. Oncoimmunology. 2020;**9**(1):1846926. DOI: 10.1080/2162402x.2020.1846926

[95] El-Khoueiry A. Atezolizumab and bevacizumab combination therapy for hepatocellular carcinoma. Gastroenterology and Hepatology (New York). 2020;**16**(3):145-148

[96] Woei-A-Jin FJSH, Weijl NI, Burgmans MC, Fariña Sarasqueta A, van Wezel JT, Wasser MNJM, et al. Neoadjuvant treatment with angiogenesis-inhibitor dovitinib prior to local therapy in hepatocellular carcinoma: A phase II study. The Oncologist. 2021;**26**(10):854-864. DOI: 10.1002/onco.13901

[97] Sarantis P, Tzanetatou ED, Ioakeimidou E, Vallilas C, Androutsakos T, Damaskos C, et al. Cholangiocarcinoma: The role of genetic and epigenetic factors; current and prospective treatment with checkpoint inhibitors and immunotherapy. American Journal of Translational Research. 2021;**13**(12):13246-13260

[98] Wang L, Sun L, Liu R, Mo H, Niu Y, Chen T, et al. Long non-coding RNA MAPKAPK5-AS1/PLAGL2/HIF-1α signaling loop promotes hepatocellular carcinoma progression. Journal of Experimental & Clinical Cancer Research. 2021;**40**(1):72. DOI: 10.1186/s13046-021-01868-z

[99] Bruix J, Qin S, Merle P, Granito A, Huang Y-H, Bodoky G, et al. Regorafenib for patients with hepatocellular carcinoma who progressed on sorafenib treatment (RESORCE): A randomised, double-blind, placebo-controlled, phase 3 trial. Lancet. 2017;**389**(10064):56-66. DOI: 10.1016/S0140-6736(16)32453-9

[100] Hindson J. T cells in NASH and liver cancer: Pathology and immunotherapy. Nature Reviews. Gastroenterology and Hepatology. 2021;**18**(6):367. DOI: 10.1038/s41575-021-00461-1

Chapter 6

Hepatocellular Carcinoma and Liver Transplantation

Umut Tüysüz

Abstract

Hepatocellular carcinoma (HCC) is the sixth most common cancer worldwide. It has the third most common cancer-related death. Here, there are different treatment options for HCC that develops on cirrhosis background. These include liver resection, liver transplantation (LT), locoregional therapy (LRT), and systemic therapy. LT is an effective treatment choice for eligible patients who provide excellent posttransplant outcomes with a low risk of HCC recurrence, especially when strict patient selection criteria and appropriate posttransplant management are applied. Different selection criteria have been proposed for LT candidates in recent years. The use of these criteria also allows for recurrence rates that can be achieved at acceptable rates. These models continue to evolve and incorporate features such as tumor biology in addition to the response to LRT as efforts to identify patient populations that may benefit more from LT by expanding access to it. Milan criteria were considered the gold standard for LT. Post-LT HCC recurrence is among the leading causes of death in patients transplanted for this indication. Posttransplant HCC surveillance is important in this regard. Early diagnosis and aggressive treatment have been proven to improve survival outcomes.

Keywords: hepatocellular carcinoma, liver transplantation, survival, recurrence, prognosis

1. Introduction

The regenerative capacity of the liver was first described in Greek mythology in the story of Prometheus. A thorough understanding of the segmental anatomy of the liver, on the other hand, was first introduced by Couinaud [1] and then by Bismuth [2]. Although the mechanism of liver regeneration is not fully understood, it has played an important role in the development of liver surgery and living donor liver transplantation (LDLT) as a result of these processes. Following the Hannover team's first demonstration of the feasibility of the innovative split-liver transplantation (SLT) in 1988, reduced-size liver transplantation and SLT were performed together in a child as LDLT in Australia by Strong using segments 2 and 3 from the mother's liver [3, 4]. OLT is the recognized optimal treatment for patients with the low-volume unresectable disease.

The first successful adult recipient LDLT was performed in Japan as left lobe and then right lobe transplantation [5, 6]. LDLT outcomes have been improving more in recent years. The concomitant organ shortage, along with concerns related to faith and ethical issues, the decrease in deceased organ donation, and increased demand for liver transplantation, has caused the need for LDLT to increase even more. There has been a continuous rise in the incidence of liver cancer and liver cancer-associated mortality and in recent decades. In 2020, it was the sixth most common cancer worldwide with a total of 905,677 new cases worldwide. It had the third most common cancer-related death with 830,180 deaths [7]. As many as 20–40% of worldwide liver transplants are for the treatment of HCC [8].

Hepatocellular carcinoma (HCC) patients are widely distributed, especially in East Asia and Africa. However, incidence and mortality have recently increased considerably in North America and Europe [9, 10]. The epidemiology of HCC has changed markedly in recent decades. While the relationship with viral hepatitis is decreasing in certain parts of the world, the relationship with alcohol and nonalcoholic fatty liver disease (NAFLD) is increasing, especially in the Western World. The median age of diagnosis in the United States is usually the sixth decade of life (60–65 in men and 65–69 in women).

HCC prevalence varies by gender and is more prevalent in men. Likewise, HCC incidence and mortality vary significantly with race and ethnicity. A higher incidence is observed in the African American and Hispanic populations [11]. Approximately 90% of HCC cases occur in the background of cirrhosis. The most common causes of cirrhosis leading to HCC in the United States are alcohol-related liver disease (ALD), NAFLD or nonalcoholic steatohepatitis (NASH), viral hepatitis B [HBV], and hepatitis C [HCV]. However, in the absence of cirrhosis, the most common cause of HCC is HBV although there has been a recent increase in HCC due to non-cirrhotic NAFLD [11]. Liver function is defined as compensated or decompensated. Decompensated liver disease is defined as jaundice, ascites, or hepatic encephalopathy regardless of Model for End-Stage Liver Disease (MELD). Stage migration describes the patient concept for whom it is necessary to make reclassification as a more advanced stage due to the changing factors even if TNM classification, the degree of liver dysfunction, and PS remain unchanged. Detection of stage migration includes progression pattern, growing or newly emerging extra or intrahepatic lesions, and newly detected vascular invasion. Liver transplantation (LT) is the treatment of choice in patients with clinically significant portal hypertension (CSPH) or significant liver dysfunction and cirrhosis if there are no medical or psychosocial contraindications.

LT is a treatment that is intended as the last option in HCC patients who still cannot be treated surgically and in impaired liver function or advanced HCC. Recently, 1100 patients per year in Europe have undergone LT due to HCC. And the annual number of new HCC cases is reported to be as high as 65,000 [12]. The introduction of direct acting antiviral therapies (DAAs) for the treatment of HCV has provided some promise in the areas of transplantation and infectious disease [13]. As a result, the number of patients listed for LT due to HCV continues to decrease. The LT perspective for HCC is parallel to the change in patients transplanted for primary liver disease. Between 2014 and 2019, the percentage of patients listed for LT due to HCV-associated HCC decreased by 22%, while the percentage of patients listed for LT due to NASH-associated HCC increased by 14.5%. NASH was the most common etiology of HCC in women listed for LT in 2019. However, although it tends to decrease in men, the most common indication for LT listing is HCV-associated HCC [14]. There is a distinct racial difference here. Compared to Caucasians and Hispanics, Black patients have high HCV associated with HCC load, which constitutes a potential obstacle for HCV treatment. On the other hand, hepatitis B virus (HBV) is the most common etiology in HCC-associated LT list among Asian patients.

After the first successful LT in 1967, the National Organ Transplant Movement established the beginning of transplantation in 1984 and organized United Network for Organ Sharing (UNOS) with a registry system to track transplant results and data [15]. LT UNOS distribution has recently taken into account multiple factors including distance of recent donor to hospital, blood type, waiting time, and severity of liver disease.

Distribution policies help reduce bias and improve post-LT outcomes. To begin with, the waiting list implemented the Child-Pugh classification system, which better emphasized the disease severity.

In 2002, the UNOS Model for End Stage Liver Disease (MELD) was launched. In 2016, the MELD-Na scoring system was introduced, which took serum sodium level into consideration. Finally, in 2023, the MELD model was corrected again by including gender and albumin level [16]. Recently, UNOS T1 (a tumor up to 2 cm) or UNOS T2 (a tumor up to 5 cm or three tumors up to 3 cm) were identified as eligible patients with non-MELD scores after a mandatory waiting period of 6 months. Here, UNOS could select the population with much better post-LT prospects among the patients with tumors that respond to treatment. To do this, UNOS is now combining alpha-fetoprotein (AFP) changes with DS data to provide exception scores to the most suitable candidates. Here, there are different treatment options for HCC that develops on cirrhosis background. These include liver resection, liver transplantation (LT), locoregional therapy (LRT), and systemic therapy. The choice of treatment or combination of therapies depends on the extent of the tumor, extrahepatic spread, macrovascular invasion, preserved liver function, and performance status (PS) [17]. LT is the only feasible curative approach in HCC patients with considerably impaired liver function. A prerequisite for the application of LT as a treatment is that the neoplasm is localized especially in the liver.

The Barcelona Clinic Liver Cancer (BCLC) staging system is recommended by American Association for the Study of Liver Diseases (AASLD) and the European Association for the Study of the Liver (EASL). This was updated in 2022 to better define the prognosis and most appropriate treatment option [17]. The BCLC staging system, which is used to determine the target population in clinical research studies, also regulates the inclusion/exclusion criteria to determine the patient profile. Clinical practice guidelines and algorithms, such as the BCLC model, indicate the most up-to-date state of scientific evidence and knowledge appropriate for each intervention. Major hepatectomy carries extreme risk in patients with cirrhosis. Specific tumor localizations can also sometimes be an obstacle to resection [18]. Large tumors are often associated with cancer-related symptoms (pain, etc.), which indicates poor outcome after resection. Upon listing for LT, if the expected waiting time exceeds 6 months, a number of treatment options are considered to prevent the tumor from progressing and being excluded from LT. Ablation, transarterial chemoembolization (TACE), and transarterial radioembolization (TARE) are the most commonly used methods for this purpose. In patients with peripheral tumor localization who were initially selected for ablation, this approach may be contraindicated due to the risk of tract seeding or adjacent organ damage (if puncture was performed without a non-tumor liver rim) [19]. The BCLC 2022 staging system version does not recommend resection for multinodular HCC within the Milan criteria. Although resection cohort studies report promising survival outcomes, prospective data are necessary to determine its effectiveness [20]. TACE should be preferred when the first-line treatment approaches for HCC (ablation or LT) are not appropriate. However, it is known that tumors exceeding 8–10 cm are associated with poor prognosis after TACE [21, 22].

This is potentially related to disruption of portal venous flow due to compression or invasion rather than the effect of major tumor necrosis. Moreover, large tumors are rarely asymptomatic. Patients with symptoms (performance status 1) have lower survival after TACE compared to asymptomatic patients [23]. In the 2022 BCLC version, BCLC stage B was divided into three groups according to tumor burden and liver function. This stage is determined as multifocal HCC that exceeds BCLC-A criteria. Here, liver function is preserved, and there are no cancer-related symptoms (PS-0) and no vascular invasion or extrahepatic spread. At this stage, the size of the tumor burden may be heterogeneous, and the prognosis is also affected by AFP levels [24]. For BCLC-0 and A, ablation should be the preferred approach if the patients are not candidates for LT. But there is not a strong cutoff value for this. An individualized patient profile can determine whether the patient would benefit from LT, systemic therapy, or TACE [22, 25]. BCLC-B stage group 1 covers well-defined HCC nodules. These patients are candidates for LT if they meet the Extended Liver Transplant criteria according to the center criteria [26–32]. A slight increase in tumor size and number provides acceptable survival outcomes. However, this may lead to a slight increase in recurrence and a decrease in long-term survival [33]. Competitive survival can be achieved with patients within Milan criteria, taking into account the reduced survival and increased risk of recurrence in patients who are allowed to progress to asymptomatic limited progression exceeding the Milan criteria [34]. Accordingly, the decision to adopt the expanded criteria is determined by the factors such as the prevalence of access to LT for other indications, and this should be comparable to the minimal results achieved for other indications.

A cutoff value of 1000 ng/dl has recently been applied as an exclusion criterion. Even if downstaging treatment induces a decrease in AFP level, there is no strong data on the reduction required or the time period to wait before LT planning. Non-MC patients with low AFP levels have better post-LT survival than those within MC but with high AFP values. AFP level intervals and UNOS exception scores are now included in the post-LT prognostic model [35]. However, patients in BCLC-B group 2 include those with preserved portal flow and defined tumor burden, and patients whose feasibility of selective access to the tumor-feeding artery was evaluated, besides the LT option. These patients are candidates for TACE. If these patients are not within the scope of either TACE or extended liver transplant criteria, systemic treatment should be recommended to ensure optimal results [36, 37]. BCLC-B group 3 patients include diffuse, extended, and infiltrative HCC covering the liver. They do not benefit from LT and TACE. Systemic treatment options should be recommended [38]. BCLC-C stage patients include the ones who are relatively fit with extrahepatic spread or vascular invasion. These patients have PS ≤ 2 and preserved liver function. They should be evaluated for systemic therapy [39]. BCLC stage D includes patients with impaired liver function and/or cancer-related symptoms (PS > 2) who do not have an LT option due to HCC burden or non-HCC factors. However, LT may be an option for patients whose tumor burden does not exceed the specified criteria.

1.1 Selection criteria for LT

Pre-LT imaging techniques identify macroscopic metastases but do not guarantee the exclusion of microscopic ones. In order to reduce the risk of unidentified micrometastasis to prevent post-LT recurrence, different selection criteria have been proposed for LT candidates in recent years. The use of these criteria also allows for recurrence rates that can be achieved at acceptable rates. The molecular profile still cannot predict the risk of recurrence, the best treatment option, and patient outcomes after successful ablation or surgery [40].

LT is an effective treatment choice for eligible patients who provide excellent posttransplant outcomes with a low risk of HCC recurrence, especially when strict patient selection criteria and appropriate posttransplant management are applied. Although cirrhotic patients who underwent liver transplantation due to HCC have the longest survival, high recurrence and short survival are often observed after early intervention. Therefore, the threshold value of the tumor burden must be well-defined [41]. Due to the strong effect of HCC recurrence on posttransplant prognosis, many criteria and scoring systems have been established for the selection of transplant candidates.

More than two decades ago, in 1996, Mazzaferro published the results referred to as the Milan criteria. They were considered the gold standard for LT. They have become the cornerstone of selection policies in HCC patients waiting for LT globally. Of course, simple and easy-to-use criteria like these have had a profound impact on survival, dramatically increasing cure rates in HCC patients receiving LT worldwide. Accordingly, there should be ≤5 cm single tumor or a maximum of three ≤3 cm tumors, and there should be no macrovascular invasion or extrahepatic spread. Here, after LT, a 4-year overall survival rate of 75% and a recurrence-free survival rate of 83% were achieved [26]. However, despite its usefulness and reproducibility advantage, it has major limitations. More importantly, there is a lack of biomarkers of the tumor that would affect the best oncological outcomes after transplantation. By including biological tumor indices, selection models go beyond the simple tumor burden.

These models continue to evolve and incorporate features such as tumor biology in addition to the response to LRT as efforts to identify patient populations that may benefit more from LT by expanding access to it [42]. The use of downstaging for this purpose has led to LT expansion efforts for HCC that exceeds the Milan criteria. Although UNOS-DS (United Network for Organ Sharing-Downstaging) has expanded LT indications for HCC patients beyond traditional MC, the outcomes of patients with tumor burden beyond UNOS-DS are still a matter of interest. Here, the upper limit of the tumor is yet to be determined [43]. Many groups recommend transplantation with results comparable to Milan for patients with larger numbers and larger tumors. The vast majority of them use radiological morphometric criteria. They represent the explant pathology that predicts the outcomes. Because of the close relationship between morphometrics and outcomes, they have become the standard treatment in HCC patients who exceed the Milan criteria. The combination of dynamic markers for wait time and response to LRT and important tumor markers allows for the successful selection of broad criteria without risking expected outcomes. After the adoption of the Milan criteria around the world, some groups emphasized the extreme restrictiveness of these criteria. The wide benefits of the original morphometric criteria also indicated excellent posttransplant outcomes. In the United States, Yao et al. proposed the University of Southern California San Francisco (UCSF) criteria in 2007 showing that expansion of the upper limit of tumor size and addition of total tumor diameter did not adversely affect outcomes, with an 80% 5-year survival for those within UCSF (single tumor ≤6.5 cm, up to three tumors ≤4.5 cm, total tumor diameter ≤ 8 cm) and poor outcomes in those outside the UCSF criteria. These criteria led to a favorable 5-year patient survival rate of 75.2% and a post-LT recurrence rate of 11.4% [44]. Here, the 4-year survival was 70% for patients in Milan criteria and 64% for patients in UCSF but outside Milan. Survival was poor in transplant recipients who did not meet both criteria. For them, the 5-year survival was only 41%. Later, in

2009, Mazzaferro et al. proposed their "Up-To-Seven Criteria" based on patients who exceeded the Milan criteria in explant pathology with a multi-inductive collaboration. Subjects are considered for OLT (orthotopic liver transplantation). These criteria include non-Milan patients without microvascular invasion (MVI). The number of nodules should not be more than seven, and the diameter of the largest nodule does not exceed 7 cm. Five-year survival was similar to patients within the Milan criteria (73.3% within Milan, 71.2% Outside Milan within Up-To-Seven), and this was referred to as the Metroticket model [45]. A morphometric selection model was also adopted by some Canadian centers. This was introduced by Toso et al. as total tumor volume (TTV). Here, HCC patient selection *via* TTV should not exceed 115 cm^3. Compared to Milan and UCSF, it further increases total inclusivity (28–53% patient increase compared to Milan criteria, and 16–26% patient increase compared to UCSF criteria). It had similar patient outcomes as Milan (beyond Milan within TTV vs. within Milan – 5-year overall survival (OS) 74 vs. 79%, 5-year recurrence-free survival (RFS) 78 vs. 80%). Broad morphometric criteria other than the Milan criteria always include more patients who would have LT and ensure survival with acceptable risk of recurrence. However, unless combined with tumor biology markers, tumor number and size alone cannot accurately predict tumor biology. Deficiencies in tumor biology limit the ability to perform risk stratification due to the gap between pathology and radiology. This limits the use of morphometric criteria alone [46, 47]. These criteria are based on the morphological characteristics of HCC. Liver imaging techniques such as contrast-enhanced computed tomography or magnetic resonance imaging are configured according to the pre-LT precision. However, they are affected by suboptimal sensitivity and heterogeneity [48]. The efficacy of these criteria in predicting acceptable disease recurrence rate and post-LT survival is based on the principle of tumor burden. The size and number of the nodules are considered to be a marker representing the presence of microvascular invasion and/or poor differentiation, which is an independent predictor of HCC recurrence. Macroscopic vascular invasion is considered to be an unacceptable risk factor for post LT. In recent years, it has been understood how microvascular invasion is associated with a high recurrence rate [49]. The diagnosis of HCC in cirrhotic individuals is often based on radiological criteria in accordance with the latest guidelines. Precise information about microvascular invasion before transplantation cannot be provided by these methods. Liver biopsy is stored in cases with nontypical imaging [37, 50]. However, although not performed routinely, histological examination provides a direct perspective on tumor grade. The expanded Toronto criteria suggested the idea of considering preoperative histology. Accordingly, LT was performed in the group of patients with no poorly differentiated neoplasm in preoperative histology from the largest nodule, no extrahepatic spread including macrovascular invasion, and no cancer-related symptoms with tumor nodules of any size and number. These expanded Toronto criteria were later confirmed by a prospective ITT study. In the Toronto study, high levels of AFP at the time of transplantation and listing were associated with poor post-LT outcomes in patients transplanted according to both within Milan and extended Toronto criteria. AFP levels and slopes appear to be appropriate prognostic indicators, and a cutoff level of 500 ng/ml was suggested as a poor prognostic factor. Sapisochin et al. showed an excellent 5-year OS outcome of 68% in patients who had transplants using AFP and tumor differentiation of any size and number beyond group criteria [51]. A number of tumor biomarkers have been proposed and validated to improve prediction of survival and recurrence outcomes. These are serum tumor and inflammatory markers [46, 47, 52, 53].

In 2018, the model known as Metroticket 2.0 was proposed. These morphological characteristics and AFP as a representative marker of microvascular invasion were created to predict HCC-specific death [30]. Dynamic changes in AFP levels are also noteworthy. In 2009, in France, it was determined that a 15 μg/l monthly increase in AFP was a poor prognostic factor in transplant recipients, and then a 27% difference in 5-year RFS was demonstrated with an upward progression of AFP values every month before LT. Survival improved in patients with lower AFP progression. However, there was no specific regulation for non-Milan patients. Nevertheless, this factor was not significant in multivariate analysis, which showed that progression of AFP was more important than morphometrics [54]. This study was subsequently confirmed by intention-to-treat (ITT). The AFP curve was crucial in predicting post-LT and waiting list in patients outside and within criteria. The 5-year ITT OS and RFS for patients with AFP < and > 15 ng/ml/month were 66.0 versus 36.7% and 92.3 versus 53.8%, respectively [55]. The ideal AFP cutoff value for AFP is <10 ng/ml, and this is an independent predictor of post-LT HCC recurrence. This rate is 50% for AFP > 10 ng/ml compared to 11% recurrence rate for AFP < 10 ng/ml.

Explant findings that considerably increase the risk of HCC recurrence include the presence of viable HCC, number of viable tumors, satellite nodules, and exceeding the Milan criteria [56]. Various AFP levels are also recommended as cutoffs for patient selection. It was stated that in Milan transplantation, AFP value >400 IU/ml was an independent predictor for survival, regardless of tumor size and number. But here, non-Milan patients were 36% [57]. It was also proven that there is a high risk of dropout from the waiting list after LRT, with the highest dropout probability at high AFP values ranging from 20 to 500 [58]. It is known that extremely high AFP levels (> 1000 ng/dl) are associated with poor outcomes in both patients undergoing LT and in listed patients. In the UCSF cohort, patients with AFP > 1000 ng/dl were shown to be strongly associated with MVI. It was emphasized that AFP > 1000 ng/dl was a strong predictor for OS and RFS. It is also known that AFP > 1000 is consistently associated with poor post-LT OS and DFS, as well as poor explant pathological features [59, 60]. Combining AFP with morphometric tumor markers is also important in selected eligible patients who exceed the criteria for LT. Toso used the combination of AFP and TTV to predict post-LT outcomes. It was later proven that patients within the TTV/AFP criteria had the same overall survival and disease-free survival rates as those within the Milan criteria [61, 62]. At the increase levels of AFP > 100 ng/dl, there is a progressive deterioration in OS and RFS [29]. After this, the AFP model combining different AFP levels and morphometric criteria was introduced. This model independently predicted well the risk of tumor recurrence and vascular invasion. The model combined tumor size (3 cm, 3–6 cm, and > 6 cm), tumor number, and AFP and had excellent ability to predict outcomes in non-Milan patients. While the model showed acceptable results in non-MC patients with AFP ≤100 ng/mL, it had a better ability to predict HCC recurrence than MC alone. In non-Milan patients with low AFP scores, the 5-year recurrence rate was 7.7% in the training cohort and 14.4% in the validation cohort. On the contrary, in non-Milan patients with high AFP scores, the rates were 46.3% and 47.55, respectively [29]. Mazzaferro up-to-7 for AFP < 200, up-to-5 for AFP 200–400, and up-to-4 for AFP between 400 and 1000 indicated that the perfect result was achieved at the lowest tumor size. This was later externally validated and accepted for the liver delivery system combining the AFP model and Metroticket 2.0 [30]. Only static AFP levels were used here. A new scoring system was subsequently developed that used dynamic AFP to predict RFS. The difference between maximum and final AFP was found to predict post-LT outcomes.

It was proven that LRT in patients with max AFP > 1000 ng/dl has similar results as those with max AFP < 1000 and 50% response, as in those with max AFP between 200 and 1000 and those with latest AFP < 200 ng/mL. It was proven that LRT in patients with max AFP > 1000 ng/dl has similar results to those with max AFP < 1000 and 50% response as those with max AFP between 200 and 1000 and those with latest AFP < 200 ng/mL. Pretransplant rapid AFP increase was reported to be a poor prognostic indicator in HCC patients undergoing LT [63].

The combination of radiologic tumor burden with AFP is important in improving the criterion decision in patients other than traditional MC. The New York/California (NYCA) scoring system, which combines AFP response with tumor size and number, demonstrated superiority to predict HCC recurrence compared to the Milan and the French AFP scoring systems. This model validated the inclusion of AFP response within the selection criteria, allowing to expand the non-Milan criteria to offer LT to patients otherwise denied LT. Importantly, this scoring system correlated the degree of AFP response with tumor differentiation and vascular invasion. This system also showed that over 85% of patients in Milan could be recategorized into low or acceptable NYCA with a 5-year RFS > 70%.

The most commonly used tumor marker is alpha-fetoprotein (AFP). It was first noticed as a diagnostic and confirmatory marker in the late 1960s and early 1970s. Disagreement over appropriate AFP increase levels resulted in a tumultuous history that could have brought an end to the use of AFP in 2001 [64]. However, the evidence regarding the benefit of AFP has recently supported its revival [65]. As a result, AFP has been shown to be useful as a prognostic marker.

AFP is strongly associated with reduced survival and pathological characteristics in patients with HCC. Serum AFP levels are also strongly associated with pathological characteristics of the tumor, such as vascular invasion and poor differentiation, and with OS and RFS [60, 66, 67]. Especially when used in conjunction with morphological criteria, the AFP level is a useful tool in identifying patients with high risk of recurrence before LT [68]. There are other biological tumor markers that are useful in non-Milan HCC patient selection. Vitamin K absence-induced protein (PIVKA-II) is one of them. It is also known as des-gamma-carboxy prothrombin. In the absence of vitamin K, it is released into the blood as abnormal prothrombin. It was identified as an HCC biomarker by Liebman et al. in 1984. It was found that patients with biopsy-confirmed HCC had a 91% increase in liver disease compared to those with metastatic cancer or chronic active hepatitis [69]. High PIVKA-II level predicts poorly differentiated tumor and MVI. PIVKA II is widely used in Asia to predict outcomes after LT, especially in the living donor liver transplant arrangement (LDLT). A multicenter Japanese study showed a 5-year RFS of 83.5% after LDLT in non-Milan patients with PIVKA II < 100 and AFP < 200, while a multicenter Korean study combined AFP with PIVKA II. It showed good results in non-Milan patients, especially in the advanced HCC subgroup and at low AFP/PIVKA II level. It was shown that the 5-year RFS in advanced HCC patients with AFP + PIVKA II < 300 was 53.4% compared to 10.1% in patients with AFP + PIVKA II > 300 [70].

Another marker is neutrophil-lymphocyte ratio (NLR). Post-LT recurrence is associated with decreased survival in HCC patients with NLR ≥5. A high recurrence rate of 62% was observed in patients with high NLR, whereas a recurrence rate of 13% was found in patients with normal NLR. Patients within Milan NLR ≥5 had a worse 5-year RFS rate than within Milan patients with normal NLR (30 vs. 81%, respectively). A much better survival rate was found in non-Milan patients with low NLR than in-Milan patients with high NLR (61 vs. 30%, respectively) [71–74].

1.2 Bridge therapies and downstaging for liver transplantation: ablation, TACE, and TARE

In patients with HCC, LDLT offers an attractive alternative to patients awaiting suitable deceased donor liver transplant (DDLT). For advanced HCC beyond MC, transplantation is more appropriate for LDLT as opposed to DDLT. The scarcity of organ distribution required for those with optimal expected survival in DDLT is a major problem.

Downstaging therapy is defined as tumor downstaging after ablation/resection or treatment strategies that reduce tumor burden for risk reduction and radical surgery including LT. Thus, the patient receives greater survival benefits from these definitive treatments. A number of studies reported similar survival rates between patients who were within the Milan criteria and those who exceeded the Milan criteria at diagnosis but were successfully downstaged after LRT. Downstaging protocols require an observational period with continued disease stability. Although the tumor upper limit suitable for downstaging is still controversial, the Milan criteria are frequently used as the final decision parameter in downstaging protocols [12]. It is unclear whether LRT is necessary for HCC and cirrhotic patients who are already within the Milan criteria, as a bridge to LT to prevent tumor progression, even though they are on the waiting list.

There are different types of LRT performed for HCC: percutaneous techniques, transarterial techniques, and stereotactic body radiation therapy (SBRT). Percutaneous techniques are generally applied to up to three tumors, each measuring up to 3 cm. Here, preserved liver functions (Child-Pugh A) and the absence of untreated coagulopathy are required. These techniques include radiofrequency ablation (RFA), microwave ablation (MWA), and percutaneous ethanol injection (PEI).

Although the most commonly used technique is RFA, PEI is preferred when the lesion is very close to the main bile duct and hollow organs such as the stomach or intestine. On the other hand, if the lesion is very close to major vessels such as the inferior Vena Cava and the main hepatic vein, there is a heat-sink effect. In this case, MWA is also applied with less sensitivity to the heat-sink effect even in slightly larger lesions.

In recent years, the use of PEI has been decreasing considerably due to the greater effectiveness of RFA [75, 76]. Cirrhotic HCC patients who are initially outside the listing criteria benefit from downstaging treatment. Approximately 40–60% of cirrhotic HCC patients who are outside the Milan criteria at diagnosis eventually meet the Milan criteria with their disease downstaged after receiving LRT [77–79]. Although there is no consensus in the literature as to whether post-LT survival rates in patients who have undergone successful downstaging are similar to those in patients who are within the Milan criteria at diagnosis, results depend on the extent of disease before downstaging treatment.

Especially if the patients who are outside the Milan criteria but within the University of California at San Francisco (UCSF-DS) (1 lesion >5 cm and ≤ 8 cm, or 2–3 lesions with at least 1 > 3 cm and ≤ 5 cm, or 4 to patients with 5 lesions, none of them is >3 cm and total tumor diameter ≤ 8 cm) during diagnosis undergo successful downstaging, they have post-LT survival similar to those within the Milan criteria at diagnosis. However, even if successful DS is performed in cases beyond the UCSF-DS criteria, they have a lower survival rate than patients within the Milan criteria [79, 80]. Moreover, LRT is also used as bridging in cirrhotic HCC patients who are on the waiting list within the Milan criteria to prevent dropping off the list or disease progression. Non-comparative studies report the dropout rate in patients without bridging treatment as 25–40% and the rate in patients without bridging treatment as

10–20%. Here, the time spent on the waiting list was determined to be 6–12 months. This is not clear for transplant waiting times of less than 6 months [41].

The most commonly used method for LRT is TACE, followed by RFA and MWA. While radiological complete response is observed in 30% of cases, only 20% of cases have pathological complete response.

LRT bridging treatment in cirrhotic HCC patients within the Milan criteria reduces neither the risk of disease recurrence after LT nor the risk of dropout from the waiting list. While a lower risk of death is observed in the first year after LT, this advantage decreases later on. Here, within the Milan criteria, there is no difference between bridging or non-bridging for 3- or 5-year overall survival after LT [81]. It is also necessary to pay attention to the management of HCC patients during the waiting period before LT. Bridging and monitoring to ensure patients remain within transplant criteria is based on HCC and underlying liver disease and the patient's fitness status. On the other hand, similar treatment is recommended for the purpose of downstaging in the subgroup of patients who are outside the transplant criteria. Indications and treatment procedures vary in centers, depending on their experience.

Frequently, TARE treatment is described to include the procedures described. In the TARE technique, radioisotope yttrium-90 absorbed into microspheres is administered percutaneously or selectively through the hepatic artery feeding the targeted tumor. Y-90 is a substance that emits short-lived beta rays and has limited tissue penetration. Microspheres in glass or resin have different sizes and numbers of beads and different specific bead activities. Before treatment, tumor mapping is performed with cone-beam CT-guided angiography and tumor stimulation is carried out with 150 MBq technetium-99 m macro-aggregated albumin. After treatment, SPECT/CT or PET/CT is performed to evaluate microsphere distribution and target mean dose in the liver and lung.

TARE methods can involve the entire liver by distributing the microspheres from the appropriate hepatic artery to the entire liver, or they can be performed bilobarly with a catheter placed in both lobes simultaneously, or segmentally or sub-segmentally in a targeted lobe or less. Apart from these, two-phase TARE is also applied to the liver lobe responsible for the disease in which partial liver atrophy and growth of the healthy liver lobe are achieved with segmental TARE. In a study involving 18 patients with ipsilateral PVTT, an 83% overall response rate was observed radiologically after TARE-DS, while 72% of the patients showed response to both tumor and thrombus (complete or partial). Partial or complete opening was observed in PVTT in 11 patients [82]. In a series of 349 patients in Mount Sinai Hospital, transplantation criteria were UNOS T2. Pathological and radiological complete response rates were 34 and 56%, respectively. Of these, 22 patients underwent LT [83]. In the study of the University of Bologna, two patients out of 63 consecutive patients experienced downstaging after TARE and underwent LT. Complete and partial response was 73%. TARE and TACE were compared in a multicenter large study. In the TARE group, progression was observed in 12.9% of patients, whereas LT was performed in 22.6% of patients. While 23.1% of them were non-Milan, complete tumor necrosis was observed in 30.8% of the patients [84]. In a randomized controlled study, TARE and TACE were compared in nonsurgical BCLC stage A and B HCC patients. Nine of the 33 patients who underwent TARE had DS, and LT was performed [85]. There are three studies on LT after bridging with TARE. Two of them reported patient outcomes after LT. One study provided details of dropout from the waiting list. In two studies, median survival after LT ranged from 46 to 69 months. The 3-year survival was 92.9%. TARE experience is limited to a few centers. The whole liver TARE procedure was rarely performed. For this purpose, repeated attempts can be made safely. Despite the limited number of reports, tumor control and response rates are high, and oncological long-term survival outcomes after LT are available. The safety profile is better and acceptable compared to systemic and other local treatments. Procedure-related complications did not lead to dropout from the waiting list.

Bridging procedures are neoadjuvant therapeutic options used to prevent patients dropping out of the waiting list and disease progression during the waiting period. Downstaging, if there is disease spread outside the Milan criteria, already shows similar LT results with tumors within the Milan criteria with this option. Classically, TACE is the treatment of choice for downstaging and bridging in HCC. However, although there is a growing trend supporting TARE, only unresectable or intermediate stage HCC is valid due to the number and size of this tumor [86, 87].

Bridge treatments are adjusted depending on the relationship of the tumor with the biliary and vascular structures, the location of the tumor, and the specific tumor number. Regarding the waiting time, the period from HCC diagnosis to LT has recently been elucidated. Moving quickly to transplant may result in transplantation in patients with more aggressive tumors. There is a risk here that the biological characteristics of tumors that are more likely to recur are not adequately tested. However, prolonged waiting time is associated with dropout from the LT waiting list, and this was reported to be 18–20% per year.

In patients undergoing LT, short waiting time (median 1.6 months) was an independent predictor of poor OS. A very short waiting period (<6 months) or a very long waiting time (>18 months) was associated with an increased risk of HCC recurrence [88, 89]. But there is a time lapse as to when patients are diagnosed, referred, and then listed at a transplant center.

Data show that, regardless of the choice of LRT, complete pathological response (cPR) and degree of tumor necrosis on explant examination are associated with improved survival and reduced recurrence [90]. The likelihood of achieving cPR is less in patients who have a short waiting time and receive more than three LRTs. The first criterion to evaluate response to treatment was the response evaluation criteria in solid tumors (RECIST) where a complete response was the disappearance of all target lesions [91]. The RECIST criteria were then "modified" to mRECIST where a complete response is the loss of any intra-tumoral arterial enhancement [92].

Milan criteria (MC) are used successfully in selecting suitable candidates for orthotopic liver transplantation (OLT). Downstaging (DS) to MC concept was first published by the University of California, San Francisco (UCSF) in 2008. Additional data have emerged supporting DS as a current approach to access OLT with excellent post-LT outcomes [80]. Traditionally, the prior DS was a prediction of gain versus biological activity of tumors exceeding MC based on response to LRT. A key component of the UCSF-DS protocol is an upper limit to tumor burden.

Management of patient with HCC on the waiting list aims to avoid disease progression. The main reason for this is to reduce the risk of developing new HCC in the remnant liver and to simultaneously treat the underlying liver cirrhosis and HCC, making LT the best treatment. However, one of the concerns in HCC is the prolonged time period between diagnosis and LT, as well as overcoming the inconsistency in the selection of LT candidates for patients requiring LT and the appropriate liver graft to identify possible patients who may benefit from this procedure, as well as LT for reasons other than HCC. There is a lack of randomized controlled trials (RCTs) evaluating neoadjuvant treatment recommendations to reduce the risk of dropout due to tumor progression. If there is no appropriate LT, the criteria will be exceeded as a result of HCC progression and the chance of treatment will be lost. If organ waiting times exceeding 6 months are anticipated, locoregional treatments (LRTs) are recommended for HCC patients for LT. In 2012, the international consensus conference UNOS reported that bridge therapy would not be beneficial for patients with T1 tumors. However, UNOS T2 lesions may benefit if the expected waiting time is 6 months or more [93]. However, most patients who receive LRT for the first time before transplantation are referred by a multidisciplinary tumor board. There are many options including trans-arterial chemoembolization, trans-arterial radioembolization, thermal ablation, resection, systemic therapy, radiation, and immunotherapy.

While 42% of LT candidates who received an HCC exception score received at least one LRT in 2003, this rate was 92% in 2018. Here, TACE is still the most utilized treatment (50% in 2018), while thermal ablation is in second place with 22%. Moreover, the use of y90 and TARE in bridge treatment has increased considerably over the time. While it was used less than 5% in 2013, this rate was 19% in 2018 [94]. Accordingly, to prevent the dropout of patients from the LT waiting list, slowing down the progression of the tumor or therapeutic options are applied as a bridge to LT. Preoperative radiological evaluations and serum alpha-fetoprotein (AFP) changes are evaluated in response to this treatment [95, 96].

2. Portal vein tumor trombosis and transplantation

Approximately 44–62.2% of HCCs have advanced vascular invasion, mainly as a form of tumor thrombosis in the portal vein [97, 98]. Once portal vein tumor thrombosis (PVTT) is observed, intrahepatic and extrahepatic metastasis, portal hypertension, jaundice, and ascites are observed in a short time. After that, the median overall survival time is only 2.7 months [99].

Three-year survival is around 5% in untreated patients or those who do not receive palliative treatment [100]. Systemic treatment is generally recommended for these patients. However, treatment including ^{125}I seeding combined with transarterial chemoembolization (TACE) has also been shown to improve overall survival in HCC patients with PVTT [101, 102]. Downstaging options for patients with PVTT and HCC include radiotherapy, systemic therapy, and multimodal treatments. There are also disadvantages here such as extensive side effects and low downstaging rate [103–105]. PVTT is found in 10–40% of HCC patients at diagnosis. Its presence indicates a poor prognosis. The presence of HCC-PVTT is considered contraindicated for LT [106–109]. Only palliative treatment is recommended. Based on the BCLC prognosis and treatment strategy algorithm, tyrosine kinase inhibitors, and immunotherapy recommendation, the estimated median overall survival is 5–19 months [17]. Three- and five-year survival rates are better than patients with segmental PVTT who receive only systemic or palliative treatment, especially those with PVTT in the first and second order portals and branches [110]. These patients also have low AFP value and low SUV-Max value by fluorodeoxyglucose-18 (FDG-18) positron emission tomography (PET). They are also patients with small tumors [111, 112]. These results demonstrate long-term survival in patients, supporting the concept of favorable tumor biology.

As a result of the dual balance in LDLT with the latest downstaging treatments and the latest successes in downstaging treatment ensuring valid benefit and equitable distribution, especially in the deceased donor scenario, there have been attempts to improve post-LT survival in HCC-PVTT with upfront downstaging. In this context, full/partial response to PVTT can be achieved with radiotherapy (stereotactic body radiation therapy [SBRT]/external beam radiation therapy [EBRT]/selective internal radiation therapy [SIRT]), transarterial chemoembolization (TACE), proton beam therapy, or systemic therapy. This also improved progression-free survival and OS. In planning for DDLT and to a lesser degree planning for LDLT, patients with HCC-PVTT may also be considered for DS before LT [113–119]. In downstaging to meet the criteria, evaluations of response to DS treatment and tumor biology features are combined [120–122]. In patients treated with TARE or TARE and TACE together or with stereotactic radiotherapy alone in the DS protocol, the 5-year OS and RFS rates are 53 and 52%, respectively. In patients who remain stable during the waiting period of the disease, the absence of loss of FDG-18 uptake on PET scan and enhancement in PVTT on CT scan is a successful indicator of DS. Advanced tumor grade (grade 3 and 4) and AFP > 400 ng/ml at diagnosis are poor prognosis factors for DS before LT [120]. The benefit of transplantation is determined as the expected survival gain with LT versus the most appropriate alternative treatment. Accordingly, the highest survival with LT is in HCC patients with advanced cirrhosis and those without extrahepatic disease (BCLC stages B, C) [123, 124]. When comparing survival in patients with HCC-PVTT undergoing LDLT, transplant benefit after downstaging with sorafenib or palliative radiotherapy alone was reported to be 23 months in 3-year survival and 34 months in 5-year survival [125]. Likewise, in two separate reports, a 5-year OS of 60% was reported after DDLT in patients with HCC-PVTT who received yttrium-90 TARE for downstaging and had a complete and ongoing radiological response with successful treatment. In contrast, this rate was 0% in non-transplant patients. The 5-year OS in transplanted HCC patients after complete radiological regression of vascular invasion with locoregional therapy was 60% [56, 126].

Since 2007, palliative treatment options have also been introduced for patients with advanced stage HCC (BCLC C). Patients with preserved liver functions (Child-Pugh A and B) and ECOG performance status (PS) 0–2 are candidates for systemic treatment. In addition, systemic treatment is recommended for cancers that show tumor progression upon locoregional therapy (LRT) or are not amenable to LRT [106, 127]. The SHARP phase 3 trial, which first established the tyrosine kinase inhibitor sorafenib as first-line treatment, changed the view of inappropriate systemic treatment in advanced HCC patients showing obvious resistance to classical chemotherapeutic agents [128]. Recently, immunotherapy has been emerging as the mainstay of systemic oncological treatment for unresectable HCC. Here, together with the establishment of evidence regarding the underlying etiology that will support hepatocarcinogenesis, which may be associated with the effectiveness of immune-based therapeutic approaches, systemic treatment may play a key role, especially for NAFLD-HCC, which is often diagnosed at an advanced stage. However, there is a need for appropriate biomarkers to predict the response to immunotherapy [129]. IMbrave 150 phase 3 study identified the combination of atezolizumab and the anti-vascular endothelial growth factor (VEGF)-A antibody bevacizumab as a new first-line treatment in advanced HCC patients who had not previously received systemic treatment. Here, a 5.8 months of improvement in median OS and a 2.6 months of improvement in PFS were observed compared to sorafenib. The OS was 19.2 months better here. One of the important features showed better preserved health quality index. Here, 69.5% of the patients were viral HCC patients. A subsequent subgroup study including nonviral HCC patients did not show any difference [130]. The KEYNOTE-240 phase III trial and the CheckMate-459 phase III trial also failed to show a survival advantage in OS and PFS [131, 132]. In fact, the latest meta-analysis of phase 3 studies showed whether OS improved in patients with unresectable HCC and those with viral HCC etiology, while noninvasive disease improved OS in patients with viral HCC etiology did not show a survival benefit in viral HCCs [133].

Ideal cutoff for AFP is independently predictive of post-LT HCC recurrence with <10 ng/ml. Compared to the 11% recurrence rate for AFP < 10 ng/ml, this rate is 50% for AFP > 10 ng/ml. Explant findings that considerably increase the risk of HCC recurrence include the presence of viable HCC, number of viable tumors, satellite nodules, and criteria greater than the Milan criteria [56].

The field of transplant oncology is rapidly developing in terms of treatment options. Immunotherapy is especially becoming widespread. For a while, ICI use before LT was considered a contraindication due to concerns about graft dysfunction or loss. However, graft loss was not noted in subsequent small retrospective studies [134, 135]. Moreover, UNOS took this further and stated that taking ICI alone, along with data on the use of immunotherapy for DS or bridge before LT, is not a contraindication for the HCC MELD update. However, despite all these data, it is of great importance to determine whether ICI and TKI or radiotherapy combination treatments would reduce post-LT HCC recurrence in patients exceeding MC, whether there would be an increase in the risk of graft dysfunction with ICI, what is the ICI termination time before LT, and what are the biomarkers in the evaluation of tumor response to treatment. In patients with advanced HCC, palliative treatments with TARE or TACE alone showed a 3-year OS of 20 and 10%, respectively [136, 137].

The REFLECT study, which compared lenvatinib with sorafenib in patients with unresectable BCLC stage B or C HCC, showed similar survival results with 13.6 and 12.3 months, respectively [138]. However, in the SARAH study, only 8 months of median OS was observed with selective internal radiotherapy (SIRT) in BCLC stage C HCC patients with locally advanced tumors [139]. The use of SIRT combined with sorafenib did not provide a statistically significant advantage in OS (14 vs. 11 months) [140]. The abovementioned palliative treatments, from downstaging to LT, achieved different survival figures in HCC patients with HCC-PVTT. Patients with locally advanced HCC and patients with PVTT without extrahepatic spread should not be categorized as having systemic disease. Targeted radiotherapy at appropriate doses results in tumor regression within the portal vein. Many patients were successfully downstaged and met the transplant criteria with this method. Although the optimal period between successful downstaging and LT is not clear, LT can be performed after 3–4 months with acceptable long-term results. In patients with suitable living donor, in LDLT regulation after downstaging, levnatinib treatment is superior to alternative treatments such as immunotherapy or TARE/SBRT alone. LT may be recommended as the only way to hope for long-term survival in patients with HCC-PVTT, despite the majority having locally rather than systemically advanced disease. These were traditionally considered suitable for palliative treatment only.

HCC may be associated with PVTT 16–30% [141]. PVTT is generally classified according to the level of portal vein involvement. There are two most commonly used classifications. In the Japanese Vp classification, Vp 0: There is no PVTT. Vp1: There is segmental tumor thrombus in the segmental portal vein. Vp2: There is tumor thrombus in the secondary order branches of the portal vein. Vp3: There is tumor thrombus in the first order branches. Vp4: There is tumor thrombus in the main portal vein and/or contralateral portal vein branch [142]. In Cheng's classification, PVTT is divided into four categories. Type I: Tumor thrombus involving segmental or sectoral portal vein branches or the part above it. Type II: Tumor thrombus involving the left/right portal vein branch. Type III: Tumor thrombus involving the main portal vein. Type IV: Tumor thrombus involving the superior mesenteric vein [143]. However, the BCLC staging system and clinical guidelines do not mention these classifications. Patients with PVTT and HCC are considered to have BCLC stage C disease. This corresponds to advanced-stage disease for which systemic treatment is usually recommended. Locoregional-based downstaging treatments play an increasingly important role for HCC patients. However, there has been no approved adjuvant treatment protocol for HCC patients with PVTT so far. Prospective multicenter controlled randomized studies are required to understand the role of LT in the intent to treatment (ITT) strategy in this group of patients. Locoregional downstaging treatments, adjuvant treatments, and their standardization are important to expand the inclusion criteria for LT. Recently, the use of immunotherapy in this field has significantly changed the treatment approach, especially in HCC patients with advanced disease. Tyrosine kinase inhibitors, vascular endothelial growth factor inhibitors, and immune checkpoint inhibitors are becoming increasingly important for the treatment of HCC [144, 145]. There is no study evaluating specific LT in patients with PVTT after downstaging treatment with immunotherapy. The use of immunotherapy in cancer patients undergoing transplantation has not been explicitly approved. Here, data regarding oncological outcomes and graft rejection outcomes associated with immunosuppressive therapy, especially after LT, are not sufficient [146, 147]. Recently, there have been a number of attempts to expand LT inclusion criteria in HCC patients, including PVTT patients. Expanded criteria are primarily accepted in the regulation made in the context of LDLT. Expanded criteria including PVTT patients is retrospective in nature. Along with the large heterogeneous patient population, there are also major deficiencies in important points such as neoadjuvant downstaging or systemic treatments. Studies with LDLT reported a lower survival rate in patients with PVTT, as well as 5-year OS rates of 57 and 48% in VP 1 and 2 patients with and without prior downstaging, respectively. Therefore, there is no consensus for downstaging strategies in patients with PVTT [112, 120, 148].

Evidence regarding the benefit of LT in patients with PVTT and HCC is limited due to the short follow-up period, small sample size, and retrospective design of the studies on the subject. However, the common results are that the prognosis after LT is poor in HCC patients with lobar PVTT. PVTT is a factor that increases the risk of mortality and recurrence after LT. HCC patients with segmental PVTT with low biological aggressiveness (such as low AFP, early grade tumor) have better results in terms of DFS and OS after LT. Although LT appears to be superior to palliative systemic treatments in patients with non-extended PVTT (Cheng's type I or Vp 1-2) and HCC, OS rates are within the recommended criteria and below 70% in patients with HCC or nonmalignant LT. This must be taken into account, especially in the context of falling off waiting lists and organ shortages around the world.

A recent study has described the experience of LDLT in HCC patients who underwent DS for PVTT with an otherwise dismal prognosis. In patients successfully downstaged after stereotactic body radiation (SBRT) and transarterial chemo- or radio-embolization (TACE or TARE) treatments, the 5-year OS and RFS were 57 and 51%, respectively. This finding was comparable to HCC patients undergoing LDLT without PVT [120].

3. Recurrence and its management

Post-LT HCC recurrence is among the leading causes of death in patients transplanted for this indication. Posttransplant HCC surveillance is important in this regard. Early diagnosis and aggressive treatment have been proven to improve survival outcomes [149, 150]. Recurrence is highly variable. HCC recurrence is rare in the first year after LT (cause of death rate in the first year is 5.3%). Likewise, post-LT occurs less frequently after 5 years. However, it is known that HCC recurrence is highest within 2–3 years after transplant [151, 152]. Recurrence time also emerges as a prognostic factor. Early HCC recurrence is associated with worse prognosis [152, 153]. Using the Milan criteria, recurrence was observed in 5.7–16% of cases. This became the benchmark for all subsequently proposed criteria. The Organ Procurement and Transplantation Network/United Network for Organ Sharing (OPTN/UNOS) records confirmed that some pretransplant factors are strongly predictive of post-LT recurrence. These include poor tumor differentiation, micro or macrovascular invasion, lymph node or extrahepatic spread, explant TNM stage T3 or T4, tumor stage > T2 after downstaging, and high AFP level [154]. The overall recurrence rate observed in a systematic review was 16%. The median time from LT to recurrence is 13 months. The most common area of recurrence is extrahepatic. According to explant pathology, 51% of the patients had LT performed outside the Milan criteria [155]. The University of California, Los Angeles (UCLA) also reported that recurrence is mainly extrahepatic. Recurrence in the liver allograft was 37.8% and had a large multinodular pattern [153]. According to these results, only liver recurrence is observed in 15–40%. Extrahepatic disease is probably due to the growth of occult metastases. Several risk factors were also identified, including dynamic and static AFP levels, neutrophil/lymphocyte ratio (NLR), AFP L3, and des gamma carboxy prothrombin. AFP response to LRT is consistently superior for post-LT outcomes [90].

Geographical and ethnic factors significantly affect recurrence. While the recurrence rate is 10% in South American studies, this rate is reported to be 21% in Asian studies. Asian and African American men have a higher recurrence rate compared to Caucasians [156]. Tumor histology provides important information in predicting the risk of recurrence. Significantly increased expression of angiopoietin-2 was demonstrated in the tumor endothelium of patients with HCC recurrence. This was not evident in hepatocytes in explant pathology. In univariate analysis, BMI, AFP level at the time of transplant, endothelial angiopoietin-2 expression, Milan criterion, Metroticket AFP score, and AFP pattern were significantly associated with recurrence. However, multivariate analysis showed that only angiopoietin-2 expression was an independent factor associated with recurrence [157].

Among the histological views evaluated, multivariate analysis revealed that immune cells were the strongest prognostic predictor of recurrence. Patients undergoing LT for HCC have a distinct immune profile that differs from that of patients transplanted for other reasons. In addition, the balance of immunosuppression may affect the risk of graft rejection, on the one hand, and the risk of HCC recurrence, on the other [158, 159].

In the early posttransplant period, a considerable but temporary increase in myeloid and B cells and a decrease in T cells and natural killer cells are observed. However, within 3 weeks, the cells return to pretransplant levels. Plasmacytoid dendritic cells increase progressively after LT and peak at 2 weeks. Patients with and without HCC show very different immune cell composition, but in transplanted patients, there is little difference in these levels in the early post-LT period between the patients who would develop recurrence and those who would not. In fact, large differences in immune subgroup cell levels exist even before transplantation. In a deeper analysis, significant T14 and T21 expansion is observed starting from 3 weeks post-LT in patients who would develop HCC recurrence [160].

The probability of recurrence in the MC group (at diagnosis) is 11.3% in the 5 years after LT and 13.3% in the 10 years after LT. However, in the DS group (at the time of LT), it is 19.1% in the 5 years and 20.6% in the 10 years. On the other hand, in patients with failed HCC, DS is 38.9% in 5 years and 41.4% in 10 years. Predictors of pre-LT recurrence here are tumor burden at transplantation, LRT count of >2, and AFP level of >20 ng/dl [42]. Early recurrence within 2 years of undergoing surgery accounts for 70% of HCC patients with recurrence, is almost incurable, and has been related to very poor survival [161].

3.1 Post-LT HCC surveillance

Post LT surveillance is very important to prescribe potential curative treatments and to identify early recurrence [162]. Evidence-based recommendations for post-LT surveillance in patients with HCC are lacking. In fact, even though close surveillance is associated with better prognosis and more applicable curative treatments [150], there is a scarcity of strong studies on its effect on LT outcomes, duration, and frequency of monitoring. Therefore, the surveillance strategy includes cross-section imaging such as contrast enhanced computer tomography (CT) or magnetic resonance imaging (MRI) for the abdomen and non-contrast CT for the lungs. If there is high clinical suspicion in other areas of metastasis, such as bone and brain, these areas are included in the examination. AFP is an effective monitoring method during surveillance. For this purpose, it is measured every 6 months. Although there is no standardization in surveillance protocols, at least 3 years of surveillance is recommended. There is no difference in RFS in patients whose scans are followed up at 3 to 6 month intervals.

UCSF recommends a surveillance strategy that uses the RETREAT score, which includes the diameter of the largest tumor in addition to the microvascular invasion, serum AFP during LT, and total tumor number in liver explant pathology [162]. Accordingly, if the RETREAT score is 0 (5-year recurrence rate is 3%), surveillance is not recommended for patients. Patients with RETREAT score 1–3 require surveillance every 6 months for 2 years. While RETREAT recommends surveillance every 6 months for 5 years in patients with a score of 4, it recommends surveillance every 6 months for 2–5 years and every 3 months for the first 2 years for patients with a RETREAT score of 5 or more.

3.2 The influence of immunosuppression on HCC

The effect of immunosuppression on recurrence after LT is also a matter of debate. Immunosuppression can inhibit the immune system's ability to detect and destroy cancer cells, which may promote tumor growth. As a result, the risk of HCC recurrence also increases. Calcineurin inhibitor (CNI) is associated with a dose-dependent increased risk of recurrence [163].

Mammalian target of rapamycin (mTOR) was found to upregulate some mutations in HCC. In such cases, mTOR inhibitors have antiproliferative and antiangiogenic effects [164]. Therefore, mTOR reduces recurrence and increases survival. The International Liver Transplantation Society, in its Transplant Oncology Consensus Conference, recommended levels of lower than 10 ng/mL for tacrolimus and lower than 300 ng/mL for cyclosporine.

Although there were concerns that DAA treatment increased the aggressiveness and recurrence of HCC, this has now been proven to be unfounded. There was even a significant reduction in the risk of death in LT in patients treated with DAA [13, 165].

Management of recurrence after LT is parallel to the management of primary LT. The clear benefit of treatment modalities with curative intent has also been demonstrated. Treatment options also vary with the location and extent of recurrence, which affects survival [43]. In one study, in cases where HCC recurrence was treated after LT, the highest 3-year survival was observed in the surgery alone group as 60%, followed by the surgical and nonsurgical combined treatment group as 37%. However, in the nonsurgical group, this rate was only 11% [153].

In a large study involving 661 patients who underwent resection for HCC, 16% of patients with recurrent HCC were listed for LT. While 63% of them eventually underwent transplantation, 23% patients were dropped out due to tumor progression [166]. Salvage LT (SLT) is another recommended curative treatment option in post-liver resection. However, long-term results are not clear. Intent to treat analysis showed that 5-year ITT OS was 69% and DFS was 60%. The SLT option is successful in 56% of patients. The results of salvage transplantation appear to be comparable to the those of primary LT for HCC, even when examined on the basis of ITT [167].

LRT may be considered as a potential treatment modality for patients with unresectable recurrent HCC after LT. Systemic therapy has limited use for post-LT recurrent HCC. Compared with supportive care, sorafenib showed a median survival of 10.6 months versus 2.2 months in this group of patients. Another multikinase inhibitor, regorafenib, is used as second-line therapy. It provides median survival rate of 13.1 versus 5.5 months [168, 169]. Capecitabine has the same safety profile as sorafenib. Compared with the best supportive care, median OS of 22 versus 7 months was observed [170].

4. Conclusions

HCC recurrence after LT is still a dreadful event, occurring in up to 20% of cases. It remains challenging to individualize risk assessments for the recurrence of HCC after liver transplantation. This is increasingly important due to the rising number of patients transplanted outside the Milan criteria with extended criteria. It might be prevented by stringent pretransplant selection criteria incorporating biological markers of aggressiveness (such as response to therapy, serum markers, and histological factors) in addition to size and number of tumors. Another strategy for improvement is the further expansion of the selection criteria. In this regard, effective perioperative adjuvant therapy based on recent developments in anticancer drugs and the refinement of posttransplant immunosuppression regimens would play a key role. Routine use of recurrence risk assessment is advised to provide tailored advice for patient selection or prioritization and an adequate individualized surveillance strategy as this predicts outcomes and prognosis. İn this context should be futher provide a framework through which to design clinical trials adjusted to the risk of recurrence and test immunosuppressive strategies or new adjuvant therapies to prevent HCC recurrence after transplantation. Several advances in this sense have been made in the last decade, allowing patients with HCC broader access to LT with more precise prediction of outcomes. In the post-LT period, surveillance should be driven by post-LT risk stratification. No adjuvant treatments after LT have been validated to prevent HCC recurrence. Within the last decade, breakthroughs in immunotherapy have greatly expanded the treatment armamentarium for HCC. However, there is still an unlit corner for HCC patients awaiting LT or after LT due to the deep concern about lethal rejection induced by immunotherapy. On the one hand, there will be an increasing number of HCC patients after immunotherapy who are bridged or downstaged to be candidates for LT, as immunotherapy is now gradually becoming a part of routine or even preferred regimens for HCC systemic therapy. There are also many patients with HCC recurrence after LT who fail to respond to other therapies, and immunotherapy may be their last option. Variation in the selection criteria for liver transplantation for HCC, from solely morphological to the incorporation of surrogate markers for the biological behaviors, the acceptable tumor burden has gradually been clarified and the patients who can be expected to benefit from this procedure can be appropriately selected. To improve the thresholds of liver transplantation for HCC, one goal is to increase the number of eligible patients. The number of deceased donors, as well as the allocation rule, would directly influence the expansion of HCC patients who are eligible for liver transplantation. In terms of the tumor burden, early tumor detection is indispensable. Further, pretransplant bridging therapy to prevent dropout due to tumor progression beyond selection criteria and downstaging to an acceptable tumor burden in those who would otherwise be excluded from candidacy would contribute to the evolution of the thresholds. The criteria of Liver transplantation for HCC continue to evolve. The transplant oncology community has increasingly understood the need to move away from size and number criteria and include surrogates of biological behavior into decision-making. It is likely that in the near future, most algorithms to decide which patients will be eligible for liver transplant will incorporate indices of tumor biology.

Conflict of interest

The author declares no conflict of interest.

Author details

Umut Tüysüz
Department of Liver Transplant Surgery, ŞiŞli Etfal Hamidiye Training and Research Hospital, Istanbul, Turkey

*Address all correspondence to: umutuysuz@gmail.com

References

[1] Couinaud C. Le Foie: Etudes anatomiques et chirurgicales. Paris: Masson Editeur; 1957

[2] Bismuth H, Houssin D. Reduced-sized orthotopic liver graft in hepatic transplantation in children. Surgery. 1984;**95**:367-370

[3] Pichlmayr R, Ringe B, Gubernatis G, et al. Transplantation of a donor liver to 2 recipients (splitting transplantation) – A new method in the further development of segmental liver transplantation. Langenbecks Archiv für Chirurgie. 1988;**373**:127-130

[4] Strong RW, Lynch SV, Hong TH. Successful liver transplantation from a living donor to her son. The New England Journal of Medicine. 1990;**322**:1505-1507

[5] Hashikura Y, Makuuchi M, Kawasaki S, et al. Successful living-related partial liver transplantation to an adult patient. Lancet. 1994;**343**:1233-1234

[6] Yamaoka Y, Washida M, Honda K, et al. Liver transplantation using a right lobe graft from a living related donor. Transplantation. 1994;**57**:1127-1130

[7] International Agency for Research on Cancer. Globocan. 2020. Available from: https://gco.iarc.fr/today/data/factsheets/cancers/11-Liver-fact-sheet.pdf

[8] Sapisochin G, Bruix J. Liver transplantation for hepatocellular carcinoma: Outcomes and novel surgical approaches. Nature Reviews. Gastroenterology & Hepatology. 2017;**14**:203-217

[9] Akinyemiju T, Abera S, Ahmed M, Alam N, Alemayohu MA, Allen C, et al. The burden of primary liver cancer and underlying etiologies from 1990 to 2015 at the global, regional, and National level: Results from the global burden of disease study 2015. JAMA Oncology. 2017;**3**:1683-1691

[10] Altekruse SF, McGlynn KA, Reichman ME. HCC incidence, mortality, and survival trends in the United States from 1975 to 2005. Journal of Clinical Oncology. 2009;**27**:1485-1491

[11] Ganesan P, Kulik LM. Hepatocellular carcinoma: New developments. Clinics in Liver Disease. 2023;**27**(1):85-102

[12] Biolato M, Galasso T, Marrone G, Miele L, Grieco A. Upper limits of downstaging for HCC in LT. Cancers. 2021;**13**:6337

[13] Singal AG, Rich NE, Mehta N, et al. Direct-acting antiviral therapy for hepatitis C virus infection is associated with increased survival in patients with a history of hepatocellular carcinoma. Gastroenterology. 2019;**157**:1253-1263.e2

[14] Puigvehí M, Hashim D, Haber PK, et al. Livertransplant for hepatocellular carcinoma in the United States: Evolving trends over the last three decades. American Journal of Transplantation. 2020;**20**:220-230

[15] Birmingham K. Thomas Starzl. Nature Medicine. 2003;**9**:10

[16] Heimbach JK. Evolution of liver transplant selection criteria and U.S. allocation policy for patients with hepatocellular carcinoma. Seminars in Liver Disease. 2020;**40**:358-364

[17] Reig M, Forner A, Rimola J, et al. BCLC strategy for prognosis prediction

and treatment recommendation: The 2022 update. Journal of Hepatology. 2022;**76**:681-693

[18] Citterio D, Facciorusso A, Sposito C, Rota R, Bhoori S, Mazzaferro V. Hierarchic interaction of factors associated with liver decompensation after resection for hepatocellular carcinoma. JAMA Surgery. 2016;**151**:846

[19] Molina V, Sampson-Dávila J, Ferrer J, Fondevila C, Díaz del Gobbo R, Calatayud D, et al. Benefits of laparoscopic liver resection in patients with hepatocellular carcinoma and portal hypertension: A case-matched study. Surgical Endoscopy. 2018;**32**:2345-2354

[20] Fukami Y, Kaneoka Y, Maeda A, Kumada T, Tanaka J, Akita T, et al. Liver resection for multiple hepatocellular carcinomas: A Japanese nationwide survey. Annals of Surgery. 2020;**272**:145-154

[21] Raoul J-L, Forner A, Bolondi L, Cheung TT, Kloeckner R, de Baere T. Updated use of TACE for hepatocellular carcinoma treatment: How and when to use it based on clinical evidence. Cancer Treatment Reviews. 2019;**72**:28-36

[22] Galle PR, Tovoli F, Foerster F, Wörns MA, Cucchetti A, Bolondi L. The treatment of intermediate stage tumours beyond TACE: From surgery to systemic therapy. Journal of Hepatology. 2017;**67**:173-183

[23] Golfieri R, Giampalma E, Renzulli M, Cioni R, Bargellini I, Bartolozzi C, et al. Randomised controlled trial of doxorubicin-eluting beads vs conventional chemoembolisation for hepatocellular carcinoma. British Journal of Cancer. 2014;**111**:255-264

[24] Akayasu K, Arii S, Ikai I, Omata M, Okita K, Ichida T, et al. Prospective cohort study of transarterial chemoembolization for unresectable hepatocellular carcinoma in 8510 patients. Gastroenterology. 2006;**131**:461-469

[25] Kloeckner R, Galle PR, Bruix J. Local and regional therapies for hepato-cellular carcinoma. Hepatology. 2021;**73**:137-149

[26] Mazzaferro V, Regalia E, Doci R, Andreola S, Pulvirenti A, Bozzetti F, et al. Liver transplantation for the treatment of small hepatocellular carcinomas in patients with cirrhosis. The New England Journal of Medicine. 1996;**334**:693-699

[27] Yao FY, Ferrell L, Bass NM, Watson JJ, Bacchetti P, Venook A, et al. Liver transplantation for hepatocellular carcinoma: Expansion of the tumor size limits does not adversely impact survival. Hepatology. 2001;**33**:1394-1403

[28] Mazzaferro V, Llovet JMJM, Miceli R, Bhoori S, Schiavo M, Mariani L, et al. Predicting survival after liver transplantation in patients with hepatocellular carcinoma beyond the Milan criteria: A retrospective, exploratory analysis. The Lancet Oncology. 2009;**10**:35-43. DOI: 10.1016/S1470-2045(08)70284-5

[29] Duvoux C, Roudot-Thoraval F, Decaens T, Pessione F, Badran H, Piardi T, et al. Liver transplantation for hepatocellular carcinoma: A model including alpha-fetoprotein improves the performance of Milan criteria. Gastroenterology. 2012;**143**:985-986

[30] Mazzaferro V, Sposito C, Zhou J, Pinna AD, De Carlis L, Fan J, et al. Metroticket 2.0 model for analysis of competing risks of death following liver transplantation for hepatocellular carcinoma. Gastroenterology. 2018;**154**:128-139

[31] Herrero JI, Sangro B, Pardo F, Quiroga J, Inarrairaegui M, Rotellar F,

et al. Liver transplantation in patients with hepatocellular carcinoma across Milan criteria. Liver Transplantation. 2008;**14**:272-278

[32] Mehta N, Bhangui P, Yao FY, Mazzaferro V, Toso C, Akamatsu N, et al. Liver transplantation for hepatocellular carcinoma. Working group report from the ILTS transplant oncology consensus conference. Transplantation. Jun 2020;**104**(6):1136-1142

[33] Kwong A, Mehta N. Expanding the limits of liver transplantation for hepatocellular carcinoma: Is there a limit? Clinics in Liver Disease. 2021;**25**:19-33

[34] Ferrer-Fàbrega J, Sampson-Dávila J, Forner A, Sapena V, Díaz A, Vilana R, et al. Limited tumour progression beyond Milan criteria while on the waiting list does not result in unacceptable impairment of survival. Journal of Hepatology. Nov 2021;**75**(5):1154-1163

[35] Mehta N, Dodge JL, Roberts JP, Hirose R, Yao FY. Alpha-fetoprotein decrease from >1000 to <500 ng/ml in patients with hepatocellular carcinoma leads to improved post-transplant outcomes. Hepatology. 2019;**69**:1193-1205

[36] Forner A, Reig M, Bruix J. Hepatocellular carcinoma. Lancet. 2018;**31**:1301-1314

[37] Galle PR, Forner A, Llovet JM, Mazzaferro V, Piscaglia F, Raoul J-L, et al. EASL clinical practice guidelines: Management of hepatocellular carcinoma. Journal of Hepatology. 2018;**69**:182-236

[38] Reig M, Darnell A, Forner A, Rimola J, Ayuso C, Bruix J. Systemic therapy for hepatocellular carcinoma: The issue of treatment stage migration and registration of progression using the BCLC-refined RECIST. Seminars in Liver Disease. 2014;**34**:444-455

[39] Bruix J, Chan SL, Galle PR, Rimassa L, Sangro B. Systemic treatment of hepatocellular carcinoma. An EASL position paper. Journal of Hepatology. 2021;**75**:960-974

[40] Singal AG, Hoshida Y, Pinato DJ, Marrero J, Nault JC, Paradis V, et al. International liver cancer association (ILCA) white paper on biomarker development for hepatocellular carcinoma. Gastroenterology. 2021;**160**:2572-2584

[41] Frankul L, Frenette C. Hepatocellular carcinoma: Downstaging to liver transplantation as curative therapy. Journal of Clinical and Translational Hepatology. 2021;**9**:220-226

[42] Halazun KJ, Tabrizian P, Najjar M, et al. Is it time to abandon the Milan criteria?: Results of a bicoastal US collaboration to redefine hepatocellular carcinoma liver transplantation selection policies. Annals of Surgery. 2018;**268**:690-699

[43] Tabrizian P, Holzner ML, Mehta N, et al. Ten-year outcomes of liver transplant and Downstaging for hepatocellular carcinoma. JAMA Surgery. 2022;**157**:779-788

[44] Yao FY, Ferrell L, Bass NM, Bacchetti P, Ascher NL, Roberts JP. Liver transplantation for hepatocellular carcinoma: Comparison of the proposed UCSF criteria with the Milan criteria and the Pittsburgh modified TNM criteria. Liver Transplantation. 2002;**8**(9):765-774

[45] Llovet M, Schwartz M, Mazzaferro V. Resection and liver transplantation for hepatocellular carcinoma. Seminars in Liver Disease. 2005;**25**(2):181-200

[46] Mehta N, Yao FY. Hepatocellular cancer as indication for liver

transplantation: Pushing beyond Milan. Current Opinion in Organ Transplantation. 2016;**21**(2):91-98

[47] Yoshizumi T, Shirabe K, Mori M. It is time to abandon the Milan criteria. HepatoBiliary Surgery and Nutrition. 2019;**8**(1):56-58

[48] Lee S, Kim SS, Roh YH, Choi JY, Park MS, Kim MJ. Diagnostic performance of CT/MRI liver imaging reporting and data system V2017 for hepatocellular carcinoma: A systematic review and meta-analysis. Liver International. 2020;**40**:1488-1497

[49] Pommergaard HC, Rostved AA, Adam R, Thygesen LC, Salizzoni M, Gómez Bravo MA, et al. Vascular invasion and survival after liver transplantation for hepatocellular carcinoma: A study from the European liver transplant registry. HPB. 2018;**20**:768-775

[50] De Gaetano AM, Catalano M, Pompili M, Marinp MG, Rodriguez Carnero P, Gulli C, et al. Critical analysis of major and ancillary features of LI-RADS V2018 in the differentiation of small (<2 cm) hepatocellular carcinoma from dysplastic nodules with gadobenate dimeglumine-enhanced magnetic resonance imaging. European Review for Medical and Pharmacological Sciences. 2019;**23**:7786-7801

[51] Sapisochin G, Goldaracena N, Laurence JM, Dib M, Barbas A, Ghanekar A, et al. The extended Toronto criteria for liver transplantation in patients with hepatocellular carcinoma: A prospective validation study. Hepatology. 2016;**64**(6):2077-2088

[52] Rosenblatt RE, Tafesh ZH, Halazun KJ. Role of inflammatory markers as hepatocellular cancer selection tool in the setting of liver transplantation. Translational Gastroenterology and Hepatology. 2017;**2**:95

[53] Taketomi A, Sanefuji K, Soejima Y, Yoshizumi T, Uhciyama H, Ikegami T, et al. Impact of des-gamma-carboxy prothrombin and tumor size on the recurrence of hepatocellular carcinoma after living donor liver transplantation. Transplantation. 2009;**87**(4):531-537

[54] Vibert E, Azoulay D, Hoti E, Iacopinelli S, Samuel D, Salloum C, et al. Progression of alphafetoprotein before liver transplantation for hepatocellular carcinoma in cirrhotic patients: A critical factor. American Journal of Transplantation. 2010;**10**(1):129-137

[55] Lai Q, Inostroza M, Rico Juri JM, Goffette P, Lerut J. Delta-slope of alpha-fetoprotein improves the ability to select liver transplant patients with hepatocellular cancer. HPB. 2015;**17**(12):1085-1095

[56] Assalino M, Terraz S, Grat M, et al. Liver transplantation for hepatocellular carcinoma after successful treatment of macrovascular invasion a multi-center retrospective cohort study. Transplant International. 2020;**33**(5):567-575

[57] DuBay D, Sandroussi C, Sandhu L, Cleary S, Guba M, Cattral MS, et al. Liver transplantation for advanced hepatocellular carcinoma using poor tumor differentiation on biopsy as an exclusion criterion. Annals of Surgery. 2011;**253**(1):166-172

[58] Mehta N, Dodge JL, Goel A, Roberts JP, Hirose R, Yao FY. Identification of liver transplant candidates with hepatocellular carcinoma and a very low dropout risk: Implications for the current organ allocation policy. Liver Transplantation. 2013;**19**(12):1343-1353

[59] Hameed B, Mehta N, Sapisochin G, Roberts JP, Yao FY. Alpha-fetoprotein level > 1000 ng/mL as an exclusion criterion for liver transplantation in patients with hepatocellular carcinoma meeting the Milan criteria. Liver Transplantation. 2014;**20**(8):945-951

[60] Hakeem AR, Young RS, Marangoni G, Lodge JP, Prasad KR. Systematic review: The prognostic role of alpha-fetoprotein following liver transplantation for hepatocellular carcinoma. Alimentary Pharmacology & Therapeutics. 2012;**35**(9):987-999

[61] Toso C, Asthana S, Bigam DL, Shapiro AM, Kneteman NM. Reassessing selection criteria prior to liver transplantation for hepatocellular carcinoma utilizing the scientific registry of transplant recipients database. Hepatology. 2009;**49**(3):832-838

[62] Toso C, Meeberg G, Hernandez-Alejandro R, Dufour JF, Marotta P, Majno P, et al. Total tumor volume and alpha-fetoprotein for selection of transplant candidates with hepatocellular carcinoma: A prospective validation. Hepatology. 2015;**62**(1):158-165

[63] Halazun KJ, Rosenblatt RE, Mehta N, et al. Dynamic α-fetoprotein response and outcomes after liver transplant for hepatocellular carcinoma. JAMA Surgery. 2021;**156**:559-567

[64] Sherman M. Alphafetoprotein: An obituary. Journal of Hepatology. 2001;**34**(4):603-605

[65] Fujiki M, Takada Y, Ogura Y, Oike F, Kaido T, Teramukai S, et al. Significance of des-gamma-carboxy prothrombin in selection criteria for living donor liver transplantation for hepatocellular carcinoma. American Journal of Transplantation. 2009;**9**(10):2362-2371

[66] Onaca N, Davis GL, Jennings LW, Goldstein RM, Klintmalm GB. Improved results of transplantation for hepatocellular carcinoma: A report from the international registry of hepatic tumors in liver transplantation. Liver Transplantation. 2009;**15**(6):574-580

[67] Todo S, Furukawa H, Tada M. Extending indication: Role of living donor liver transplantation for hepatocellular carcinoma. Liver Transplantation. 2007;**13**(11 Suppl. 2):S48-S54

[68] Burra P, Giannini EG, Caraceni P, Ginanni Corradini S, Rendina M, Volpes R, et al. Specific issues concerning the management of patients on the waiting list and after liver transplantation. Liver International. 2018;**38**:1338-1362

[69] Liebman HA, Furie BC, Tong MJ, Blanchard RA, Lo KJ, Lee SD, et al. Desgammacarboxy (abnormal) prothrombin as a serum marker of primary hepatocellular carcinoma. The New England Journal of Medicine. 1984;**310**(22):1427-1431

[70] Lee HW, Song G-W, Lee S-G, Kim JM, Joh J-W, Han DH, et al. Patient selection by tumor markers in liver transplantation for advanced hepatocellular carcinoma. Liver Transplantation: Official Publication of the American Association for the Study of Liver Diseases and the International Liver Transplantation Society. 2018;**24**(9):1243-1251

[71] Halazun KJ, Hardy MA, Rana AA, Woodland DC, Luyten EJ, Mahadev S, et al. Negative impact of neutrophil-lymphocyte ratio on outcome after liver transplantation for hepatocellular carcinoma. Annals of Surgery. 2009;**250**(1):141-151

[72] Okamura Y, Sugiura T, Ito T, Yamamoto Y, Ashida R, Mori K, et al. Neutrophil to lymphocyte ratio as an indicator of the malignant behaviour of

hepatocellular carcinoma. The British Journal of Surgery. 2016;**103**(7):891-898

[73] Yoshizumi T, Ikegami T, Yoshiya S, Motomura T, Mano Y, Muto J, et al. Impact of tumor size, number of tumors and neutrophil-to-lymphocyte ratio in liver transplantation for recurrent hepatocellular carcinoma. Hepatology Research: The Official Journal of the Japan Society of Hepatology. 2013;**43**(7):709-716

[74] Templeton AJ, McNamara MG, Šeruga B, Vera-Badillo FE, Aneja P, Ocaña A, et al. Prognostic role of neutrophil-to-lymphocyte ratio in solid tumors: A systematic review and meta-analysis. Journal of the National Cancer Institute. 2014;**106**(6):dju124

[75] Jiang G, Ling S, Zhan Q, Zhuang L, Xu X. Downstaging treatment for patients with hepatocelluar carcinoma before transplantation. Transplantation Reviews (Orlando, Fla.). 2021;**35**:100606

[76] Cardarelli-Leite L, Hadjivassiliou A, Klass D, et al. Current locoregional therapies and treatment strategies in hepatocellular carcinoma. Current Oncology. 2020;**27**(Suppl. 3):S144-S151

[77] Murali AR, Romero-Marrero C, Miller C, et al. Predictors of successful downstaging of hepatocellular carcinoma outside Milan criteria. Transplantation. 2016;**100**:2391-2397

[78] Kardashian A, Florman SS, Haydel B, et al. Liver transplantation outcomes in a U.S. multicenter cohort of 789 patients with hepatocellular carcinoma presenting beyond Milan criteria. Hepatology. 2020;**6**:2014-2028

[79] Degroote H, Piñero F, Costentin C, et al. International study on the outcome of locoregional therapy for liver transplant in hepatocellular carcinoma beyond Milan criteria. JHEP Reports. 2021;**3**:100331

[80] Yao FY, Kerlan RK Jr, Hirose R, et al. Excellent outcome following down-staging of hepatocellular carcinoma prior to liver transplantation: An intention-to-treat analysis. Hepatology. 2008;**48**:819-827

[81] Kostakis LD, Dimitrokallis N. Bridging locoregional treatment prior to liver transplantation for cirrhotic patients with hepatocellular carcinoma within the Milan criteria: A systematic review and metaanalysis. Annals of Gastroenterology. 2023;**36**:449-458

[82] Pracht M, Edeline J, Lenoir L, Latournerie M, Mesbah H, Audrain O, et al. Lobar HCC with ipsilateral portal vein tumor thrombosis treated with yttrium-90 glass microsphere radioembolization: Preliminary results. International Journal of Hepatology. 2013;**2013**:827649

[83] Labgaa I, Tabrizian P, Titano J, Kim E, Thung SN, Florman S, et al. Feasibility and safety of LT or resection after transarterial radioembolization with yttrium-90 for unresectable HCC. HPB: The Official Journal of the International Hepato Pancreato Biliary Association. 2019;**21**:1497-1504

[84] Mehta N, Frenette C, Tabrizian P, Hoteit M, Guy J, Parikh N, et al. Downstaging outcomes for HCC: Results from the multicenter evaluation of reduction in tumor size before LT (MERITS-LT) consortium. Gastroenterology. 2021;**161**:1502-1512

[85] Dhondt E, Lambert B, Hermie L, Huyck L, Vanlangenhove P, Geerts A, et al. ^{90}Y radioembolization versus drug-eluting bead chemoembolization for unresectable HCC: Results from the

TRACE phase II randomized controlled trial. Radiology. 2022;**303**:699-710

[86] El Fouly A, Ertle J, El Dorry A, Shaker MK, Dechêne A, Abdella H, et al. In intermediate stage HCC: Radioembolization with yttrium 90 or chemoembolization? Liver International. 2015;**35**:627-635

[87] Lobo L, Yakoub D, Picado O, Ripat C, Pendola F, Sharma R, et al. Unresectable HCC: Radioembolization versus chemoembolization: A systematic review and meta-analysis. CardioVascular and Interventional Radiology. 2016;**39**:1580-1588

[88] Halazun KJ, Patzer RE, Rana AA, et al. Standing the test of time: Outcomes of a decade of prioritizing patients with hepatocellular carcinoma, results of the UNOS natural geographic experiment. Hepatology. 2014;**60**:1957-1962

[89] Mehta N, Heimbach J, Lee D, et al. Wait time of less than 6 and greater than 18 months predicts hepatocellular carcinoma recurrence after liver transplantation: Proposing a wait time "sweet spot". Transplantation. 2017;**101**:2071-2078

[90] DiNorcia J, Florman SS, Haydel B, et al. Pathologic response to pretransplant locoregional therapy is predictive of patient outcome after liver transplantation for hepatocellular carcinoma: Analysis from the US multicenter HCC transplant consortium. Annals of Surgery. 2020;**271**:616-624

[91] Therasse P, Arbuck SG, Eisenhauer EA, et al. New guidelines to evaluate the response to treatment in solid tumors. European organization for research and treatment of cancer, National Cancer Institute of the United States, National Cancer Institute of Canada. Journal of the National Cancer Institute. 2000;**92**:205-216

[92] Lencioni R, Llovet JM. Modified RECIST (mRECIST) assessment for hepatocellular carcinoma. Seminars in Liver Disease. 2010;**30**:52-60

[93] Clavien PA, Lesurtel M, Bossuyt PM, et al. Recommendations for liver transplantation for hepatocellular carcinoma: An international consensus conference report. The Lancet Oncology. 2012;**13**:e11-e22

[94] Kwong AJ, Ghaziani TT, Yao F, et al. National trends and waitlist outcomes of locoregional therapy among liver transplant candidates with hepatocellular carcinoma in the United States. Clinical Gastroenterology and Hepatology. 2022;**20**:1142-1150.e4

[95] Morris PD, Laurence JM, Yeo D, et al. Can response to locoregional therapy help predict long-term survival after liver transplantation for hepatocellular carcinoma? A systematic review. Liver Transplantation. 2017;**23**:375-385

[96] Lai Q, Avolio AW, Graziadei I, et al. Alpha-fetoprotein and modified response evaluation criteria in solid tumors progression after locoregional therapy as predictors of hepatocellular cancer recurrence and death after transplantation. Liver Transplantation. 2013;**19**:1108-1118

[97] Wei X, Jiang Y, Zhang X, et al. Neoadjuvant three-dimensional conformal radiotherapy for resectable hepatocellular carcinoma with portal vein tumor thrombus: A randomized, open-label, multicenter controlled study. Journal of Clinical Oncology. 2019;**37**(24):2141-2151

[98] Liu PH, Huo TI, Miksad RA. Hepatocellular carcinoma with portal vein tumor involvement: Best management strategies. Seminars in Liver Disease. 2018;**38**(3):242-251

[99] Pawarode A, Voravud N, Sriuranpong V, Kullavanijaya P, Patt YZ. Natural history of untreated primary hepatocellular carcinoma: A retrospective study of 157 patients. American Journal of Clinical Oncology. 1998;**21**(4):386-391

[100] Lee YH, Hsu CY, Huang YH, et al. Vascular invasion in hepatocellular carcinoma: prevalence, determinants and prognostic impact. Journal of Clinical Gastroenterology. 2014;**48**(8):734-741

[101] Sun H, Zhang M, Liu R, Liu Y, Hou Y, Wu C. Endovascular implantation of 125I seed combined with transcatheter arterial chemoembolization for unresectable hepatocellular carcinoma. Future Oncology. 2018;**14**(12):1165-1176

[102] Hu HT, Luo JP, Cao GS, et al. Hepatocellular carcinoma with portal vein tumor thrombus treated with transarterial chemoembolization and sorafenib vs.125Iodine implantation. Frontiers in Oncology. 2021;**11**:806907

[103] Zeng ZC, Tang ZY, Fan J, et al. A comparison of chemoembolization combination with and without radiotherapy for unresectable hepatocellular carcinoma. Cancer Journal. 2004;**10**(5):307-316

[104] Zhu XD, Huang C, Shen YH, et al. Downstaging and resection of initially unresectable hepatocellular carcinoma with tyrosine kinase inhibitor and anti-PD-1 antibody combinations. Liver Cancer. 2021;**10**(4):320-329

[105] Lee IJ, Kim JW, Han KH, et al. Concurrent chemoradiotherapy shows long-term survival after conversion from locally advanced to resectable hepatocellular carcinoma. Yonsei Medical Journal. 2014;**55**(6):1489-1497

[106] European Association for the Study of the Liver. Electronic address EEE, European association for the study of the L. EASL clinical practice guidelines: Management of hepatocellular carcinoma. Journal of Hepatology. 2018;**69**(1):182-236

[107] Heimbach JK, Kulik LM, Finn RS, et al. AASLD guidelines for the treatment of hepatocellular carcinoma. Hepatology. 2018;**67**(1):358-380

[108] Vogel A, Martinelli E, clinicalguidelines@esmo.org EGCEa, Committee EG. Updated treatment recommendations for hepatocellular carcinoma (HCC) from the ESMO clinical practice guidelines. Annals of Oncology. 2021;**32**(6):801-805

[109] Bruix J, Reig M, Sherman M. Evidence-based diagnosis, staging, and treatment of patients with hepatocellular carcinoma. Gastroenterology. 2016;**150**(4):835-853

[110] Japan LCSGo. The General Rules for the Clinical and Pathological Study of Primary Liver Cancer. 2nd ed. Tokyo, Japan: Kanehara & Co. Ltd; 2003

[111] Lee KW, Suh SW, Choi Y, et al. Macrovascular invasion is not an absolute contraindication for living donor liver transplantation. Liver Transplantation. 2017;**23**(1):19-27

[112] Choi HJ, Kim DG, Na GH, et al. The clinical outcomes of patients with portal vein tumor thrombi after living donor liver transplantation. Liver Transplantation. 2017;**23**(8):1023-1031

[113] Xi M, Zhang L, Zhao L, et al. Effectiveness of stereotactic body radiotherapy for hepatocellular carcinoma with portal vein and/or inferior vena cava tumor thrombosis. PLoS One. 2013;**8**(5):e63864

[114] Kang J, Nie Q, Du R, et al. Stereotactic body radiotherapy combined

with transarterial chemoembolization for hepatocellular carcinoma with portal vein tumor thrombosis. Molecular and Clinical Oncology. 2014;**2**(1):43-50

[115] Ding X, Sun W, Li W, et al. Transarterial chemoembolization plus lenvatinib versus transarterial chemoembolization plus sorafenib as first-line treatment for hepatocellular carcinoma with portal vein tumor thrombus: A prospective randomized study. Cancer. 2021;**127**(20):3782-3793

[116] Abouchaleh N, Gabr A, Ali R, et al. ^{90}Y radioembolization for locally advanced hepatocellular carcinoma with portal vein thrombosis: Long-term outcomes in a 185-patient cohort. Journal of Nuclear Medicine. 2018;**59**(7):1042-1048

[117] Choi HS, Kang KM, Jeong BK, et al. Effectiveness of stereotactic body radiotherapy for portal vein tumor thrombosis in patients with hepatocellular carcinoma and underlying chronic liver disease. Asia-Pacific Journal of Clinical Oncology. 2021;**17**(3):209-215

[118] Chen CL, Ong AD, Cheng JY, et al. Proton beam therapy to bridge or downstage locally advanced hepatocellular carcinoma to living donor liver transplantation. Hepatobiliary Surgery and Nutrition. 2022;**11**(1):103-111

[119] Zhang XF, Lai L, Zhou H, et al. Stereotactic body radiotherapy plus transcatheter arterial chemoembolization for inoperable hepatocellular carcinoma patients with portal vein tumour thrombus: A meta-analysis. PLoS One. 2022;**17**(5):e0268779

[120] Soin AS, Bhangui P, Kataria T, et al. Experience with LDLT in patients with hepatocellular carcinoma and portal vein tumor thrombosis postdownstaging. Transplantation. 2020;**104**(11):2334-2345

[121] Jeong Y, Shin MH, Yoon SM, et al. Liver transplantation after transarterial chemoembolization and radiotherapy for hepatocellular carcinoma with vascular invasion. Journal of Gastrointestinal Surgery. 2017;**21**(2):275-283

[122] Bhatti ABH, Naqvi W, Khan NY, et al. Living donor liver transplantation for advanced hepatocellular carcinoma including macrovascular invasion. Journal of Cancer Research and Clinical Oncology. 2022;**148**(1):245-253

[123] Vitale A, Volk M, Cillo U. Transplant benefit for patients with hepatocellular carcinoma. World Journal of Gastroenterology. 2013;**19**(48): 9183-9188

[124] Vitale A, Morales RR, Zanus G, et al. Barcelona clinic liver cancer staging and transplant survival benefit for patients with hepatocellular carcinoma: A multicentre, cohort study. The Lancet Oncology. 2011;**12**(7):654-662

[125] ILTS. Virtual international congress of ILTS, ELITA and LICAGE, digital event, May 5-8, 2021. Transplantation. 2021;**105**(8S Suppl. 1):1-190

[126] Serenari M, Cappelli A, Cucchetti A, et al. Deceased donor liver transplantation after radioembolization for hepatocellular carcinoma and portal vein tumoral thrombosis: A pilot study. Liver Transplantation. 2021;**27**(12):1758-1766

[127] Llovet JM, Kelley RK, Villanueva A, Singal AG, Pikarsky E, Roayaie S, et al. Hepatocellular carcinoma. Nature Reviews Disease Primers. 2021;**7**(1):6

[128] Llovet JM, Ricci S, Mazzaferro V, Hilgard P, Gane E, Blanc J-F, et al. Sorafenib in advanced hepatocellular carcinoma. The New England Journal of Medicine. 2008;**359**(4):378-390

[129] Roderburg C, Wree A, Demir M, Schmelzle M, Tacke F. The role of the innate immune system in the development and treatment of hepatocellular carcinoma. Hepatic. Oncologia. 2020;7(1):HEP17

[130] Finn RS, Qin S, Ikeda M, Galle PR, Ducreux M, Kim T-Y, et al. IMbrave150: Updated overall survival (OS) data from a global, randomized, open-label phase III study of atezolizumab (atezo) + bevacizumab (bev) versus sorafenib (sor) in patients (pts) with unresectable hepatocellular carcinoma (HCC). JCO. 2021;**39**(Suppl. 3):267

[131] Finn RS, Ryoo B-Y, Merle P, Kudo M, Bouattour M, Lim HY, et al. Pembrolizumab as second-line therapy in patients with advanced hepatocellular carcinoma in KEYNOTE-240: A randomized, double-blind, phase III trial. Journal of Clinical Oncology: Official Journal of the American Society of Clinical Oncology. 2020;**38**(3):193-202

[132] Yau T, Park JW, Finn RS, Cheng A-L, Mathurin P, Edeline J, et al. Check-mate 459: A randomized, multi-center phase III study of nivolumab (NIVO) vs sorafenib (SOR) as first-line (1L) treatment in patients (pts) with advanced hepatocellular carcinoma (aHCC). Annals of Oncology. 2019;**30**:v874-v875

[133] Pfister D, Núñez NG, Pinyol R, Govaere O, Pinter M, Szydlowska M, et al. NASH limits anti-tumour surveillance in immunotherapy-treated HCC. Nature. Apr 2021;**592**(7854):450-456

[134] Qiao ZY, Zhang ZJ, Lv ZC, et al. Neoadjuvant programmed cell death 1 (PD-1) inhibitor treatment in patients with hepatocellular carcinoma before liver transplant: A cohort study and literature review. Frontiers in Immunology. 2021;**12**:653437

[135] Tabrizian P, Florman SS, Schwartz ME. PD-1 inhibitor as bridge therapy to liver transplantation? American Journal of Transplantation. 2021;**21**(5):1979-1980

[136] Spreafico C, Sposito C, Vaiani M, et al. Development of a prognostic score to predict response to Yttrium-90 radioembolization for hepatocellular carcinoma with portal vein invasion. Journal of Hepatology. 2018;**68**(4):724-732

[137] Lee JM, Jang BK, Lee YJ, et al. Survival outcomes of hepatic resection compared with transarterial chemoembolization or sorafenib for hepatocellular carcinoma with portal vein tumor thrombosis. Clinical and Molecular Hepatology. 2016;**22**(1):160-167

[138] Kudo M, Finn RS, Qin S, et al. Lenvatinib versus sorafenib in first-line treatment of patients with unresectable hepatocellular carcinoma: A randomised phase 3 non-inferiority trial. Lancet. 2018;**391**(10126):1163-1173

[139] Vilgrain V, Pereira H, Assenat E, et al. Efficacy and safety of selective internal radiotherapy with yttrium-90 resin microspheres compared with sorafenib in locally advanced and inoperable hepatocellular carcinoma (SARAH): An open-label randomised controlled phase 3 trial. The Lancet Oncology. 2017;**18**(12):1624-1636

[140] Ricke J, Klumpen HJ, Amthauer H, et al. Impact of combined selective internal radiation therapy and sorafenib on survival in advanced hepatocellular carcinoma. Journal of Hepatology. 2019;**71**(6):1164-1174

[141] Khan AR, Wei X, Xu X. Portal vein tumor thrombosis and hepatocellular carcinoma - the changing tides.

Journal of Hepatocellular Carcinoma. 2021;**8**:1089-1115

[142] Kudo M. Management of hepatocellular carcinoma in Japan as a world-leading model. Liver Cancer. 2018;**7**(2):134-147

[143] Shi J, Lai EC, Li N, et al. Surgical treatment of hepatocellular carcinoma with portal vein tumor thrombus. Annals of Surgical Oncology. 2010;**17**(8):2073-2080

[144] Finn RS, Qin S, Ikeda M, et al. Atezolizumab plus bevacizumab in unresectable hepatocellular carcinoma. The New England Journal of Medicine. 2020;**382**(20):1894-1905

[145] Foerster F, Gairing SJ, Ilyas SI, et al. Emerging immunotherapy for HCC: A guide for hepatologists. Hepatology. 2022;**75**(6):1604-1626

[146] d'Izarny-Gargas T, Durrbach A, Zaidan M. Efficacy and tolerance of immune checkpoint inhibitors in transplant patients with cancer: A systematic review. American Journal of Transplantation : Official Journal of the American Society of Transplantation and the American Society of Transplant Surgeons. 2020;**20**(9):2457-2465

[147] Portuguese AJ, Tykodi SS, Blosser CD, et al. Immune checkpoint inhibitor use in solid organ transplant recipients: A systematic review. Journal of the National Comprehensive Cancer Network. 2022;**20**(4):406-416 e11

[148] Llovet JM, Pavel M, Rimola J, et al. Pilot study of living donor liver transplantation for patients with hepatocellular carcinoma exceeding Milan criteria (Barcelona clinic liver cancer extended criteria). Liver Transplantation. 2018;**24**(3):369-379

[149] Roh YN, David Kwon CH, Song S, Shin M, Man Kim J, Kim S, et al. The prognosis and treatment outcomes of patients with recurrent hepatocellular carcinoma after liver transplantation. Clinical Transplantation. 2014;**28**:141-147

[150] Lee DD, Sapisochin G, Mehta N, Gorgen A, Musto KR, Hajda H, et al. Surveillance for HCC after liver transplantation: Increased monitoring may yield aggressive treatment options and improved postrecurrence survival. Transplantation. 2020;**104**:2105-2112

[151] Daniel KE, Eickhoff J, Lucey MR. Why do patients die after a liver transplantation? Clinical Transplantation. 2017;**31**:e12906

[152] Verna EC, Patel YA, Aggarwal A, Desai AP, Frenette C, Pillai AA, et al. Liver transplantation for hepatocellular carcinoma: Management after the transplant. American Journal of Transplantation. 2020;**20**:333-347

[153] Bodzin AS, Lunsford KE, Markovic D, Harlander-Locke MP, Busuttil RW, Agopian VG. Predicting mortality in patients developing recurrent hepatocellular carcinoma after liver transplantation: Impact of treatment modality and recurrence characteristics. Annals of Surgery. 2017;**266**:118-125

[154] Harper AM, Edwards E, Washburn WK, Heimbach J. An early look at the organ procurement and transplantation network explant pathology form data. Liver Transplantation. 2016;**22**:757-764

[155] De'Angelis N, Landi F, Carra MC, Azoulay D. Managements of recurrent hepatocellular carcinoma after liver transplantation: A systematic review. World Journal of Gastroenterology. 2015;**21**:11185-11198

[156] Bzeizi KI, Abdullah M, Vidyasagar K, Alqahthani SA, Broering D.

Hepatocellular carcinoma recurrence and mortality rate post liver transplantation: Meta-analysis and systematic review of real-world evidence. Cancers. 2022;**14**:5114

[157] Lasagni S, Leonardi F, Pivetti A, Di Marco L, Ravaioli F, Serenari M, et al. Endothelial angiopoietin-2 overexpression in explanted livers identifies subjects at higher risk of recurrence of hepatocellular carcinoma after liver transplantation. Frontiers in Oncology. 2022;**12**:960808

[158] Qu WF, Tian MX, Lu HW, Zhou YF, Liu WR, Tang Z, et al. Development of a deep pathomics score for predicting hepatocellular carcinoma recurrence after liver transplantation. Hepatology International. 2023;**17**:927-941

[159] Li CX, Ling CC, Shao Y, Xu A, Li XC, Ng KTP, et al. CXCL10/CXCR3 signaling mobilized-regulatory T cells promote liver tumor recurrence after transplantation. Journal of Hepatology. 2016;**65**:944-952

[160] Wei X, Xie W, Yin W, Yang M, Khan AR, Su R, et al. Prediction of tumor recurrence by distinct immunoprofiles in liver transplant patients based on mass cytometry. American Journal of Cancer Research. 2022;**12**:4160-4176

[161] Zheng J, Kuk D, Gönen M, Balachandran VP, Kingham TP, Allen PJ, et al. Actual 10-year survivors after resection of hepatocellular carcinoma. Annals of Surgical Oncology. 2017;**24**(5):1358-1366

[162] Mehta N, Heimbach J, Harnois DM, et al. Validation of a risk estimation of tumor recurrence after transplant (RETREAT) score for hepatocellular carcinoma recurrence after liver transplant. JAMA Oncology. 2017;**3**:493-500

[163] Rodríguez-Perálvarez M, Tsochatzis E, Naveas MC, et al. Reduced exposure to calcineurin inhibitors early after liver transplantation prevents recurrence of hepatocellular carcinoma. Journal of Hepatology. 2013;**59**:1193-1199

[164] Matter MS, Decaens T, Andersen JB, et al. Targeting the mTOR pathway in hepatocellular carcinoma: Current state and future trends. Journal of Hepatology. 2014;**60**:855-865

[165] Singal AG, Rich NE, Mehta N, et al. Direct-acting antiviral therapy not associated with recurrence of hepatocellular carcinoma in a multicenter North American cohort study. Gastroenterology. 2019;**156**:1683-1692.e1

[166] Tabrizian P, Jibara G, Shrager B, et al. Recurrence of hepatocellular cancer after resection: Patterns, treatments, and prognosis. Annals of Surgery. 2015;**261**:947-955

[167] de Haas RJ, Lim C, Bhangui P, et al. Curative salvage liver transplantation in patients with cirrhosis and hepatocellular carcinoma: An intention-to-treat analysis. Hepatology. 2018;**67**:204-215

[168] Ravaioli M, Cucchetti A, Pinna AD, et al. The role of metronomic capecitabine for treatment of recurrent hepatocellular carcinoma after liver transplantation. Scientific Reports. 2017;**7**:11305

[169] Zheng SS, Xu X, Wu J, Chen J, Wang WL, Zhang M, et al. Liver transplantation for hepatocellular carcinoma: Hangzhou experiences. Transplantation. 2008;**85**:1726-1732

[170] Takada Y, Ito T, Ueda M, Sakamoto S, Haga H, Maetani Y, et al. Living donor liver transplantation for patients with HCC exceeding the Milan criteria: A proposal of expanded criteria. Digestive Diseases. 2007;**25**:299-302

Chapter 7

Hepatocellular Carcinoma: Recent Advances in Curative Liver Resection

Nguyen Hai Nam

Abstract

Hepatocellular carcinoma is the third leading cause of cancer mortality and the sixth most common cancer worldwide, posing a serious global health burden. Liver resection (LR) represents the main form of curative treatment, and it is constantly evolving, along with massive progress in the last 20 years in order to improve the safety of hepatectomy and to broaden the indication of LR. This chapter highlights the recent advances in the surgical management of HCC, including (1) the optimization of future liver remnant (FLR) with portal vein embolization, associating liver partition and portal vein ligation for staged hepatectomy and radiological simultaneous portohepatic vein embolization, (2) the advantages of anatomic LR compared to non-anatomic LR, (3) the minimal invasive liver surgery (MILS) approach via laparoscopic and robotic LR, (4) simulation as well as navigation with three-dimensional liver reconstruction and simulated LR, and application of fluorescence imaging, (5) the utilization of new parenchymal transection devices, and (6) liver transplantation (LT) versus LR. With a deeper understanding of segmental liver anatomy, assistance from simulation and navigation system, advances in FLR optimization, MILS, new parenchymal transection devices, and LT, liver surgeons should tailor the surgical plan according to each individual to achieve the best outcome for patients.

Keywords: hepatocellular carcinoma, hepatectomy, optimization of future liver remnant, anatomic liver resection, minimal invasive approach, simulation and navigation, new parenchymal transection devices

1. Introduction

Liver cancer represents one of the leading solid malignancies and the most common cause of cancer-related death. Among them, hepatocellular carcinoma (HCC) constitutes more than 90% of the primary liver tumors, with 840.000 newly diagnosed cases and over 780.000 deaths per year [1]. As the third leading cause of cancer mortality and the sixth most common cancer across the world, HCC poses a serious global health burden and results in a significant matter of disease concern [2]. At present, liver transplantation (LT), local tumor ablation (LTA), and liver resection (LR) represent the three main forms of curative options for HCC. Unfortunately,

 IntechOpen

due to the severe liver graft shortage, the risk of withdrawal from the lengthy waiting list due to tumor progression, and the stringent selection criteria, only a humble fragment of HCC patients can benefit from LT. In the same circumstances, LTA faces restrictions in its application caused by location challenges (subdiaphragmatic or subcapsular tumor), large tumor diameter (more than three cm), and close vicinity to structure (vascular, biliary, and organ). Thus, LR remains the backbone of curative therapy thanks to its flexible indication and its available facilities. The five years overall survival in HCC patients who achieve curative treatment with LR reaches 60–80% which is significant better and more promising as opposed to unresectable HCC [3]. Given its importance, in the last 20 years, LR is extendedly indicated in a more advanced stage and continues to be ameliorated with massive progress in safety and in widened indication.

In this chapter, we highlight the recent advances in the surgical management of HCC including (1) the optimization of the future liver remnant, (2) the advantages of anatomic resection compared to non-anatomic resection, (3) the minimal invasive approach via laparoscopic and robotic LR, (4) simulation and navigation in LR, and (5) the utilization of new parenchymal transection devices.

2. Advances in surgical management of HCC

2.1 Optimization of the predicted insufficient future liver remnant

The post-hepatectomy liver failure (PHLF) due to the insufficient future liver remnant (FLR) remains a critical concern in hepatectomy when the indication of major LR is essential for curative purposes. In general, a minimum FLR of 30% of the total liver volume (TLV) is a safe frontier for patients with normal liver, whereas preservation of 40–50% of TLV is imperative in case of chronic liver disease such as hepatic fibrosis or steatosis and cholestasis [4, 5]. Therefore, various strategies have been proposed to improve the resectability rate by achieving adequate compensatory liver hypertrophy.

2.1.1 Portal vein embolization (PVE)

PVE was initially introduced by the Japanese Professor Makuuchi in 1990 to minimize the risk of PHLF in patients who underwent major LR due to hilar cholangiocarcinoma [6]. The essential core behind this technique is to stimulate the enlargement of FLR by embolizing the portal vein (PV) of the tumor-bearing hepatic lobe before LR. Administration of embolic agents (such as polyvinyl alcohol particles, microspheres, gel foam, N-butyl cyanoacrylate glue, or sodium tetradecyl sulfate foam with or without combination coils/plugs) will decrease the targeted portal vascular flow by creating PV occlusion and then consequently promote hypertrophy of the non-embolized hepatic lobe via mirror liver regeneration following resection. The ultimate goal of successful PVE consists of distal PV blockage to prevent intrahepatic collaterals as well as proximal PV occlusion to stop the venous inflow in the targeted hepatic segments. This strategy has been recognized as a powerful solution for inadequate FLR modulation. The access of the targeted PV can be achieved via one of the four following approaches: the percutaneous transjugular and the intraoperative transileocolic venous approaches are clinically less preferred due to their invasiveness and the requirement of anesthesia support, whereas the transhepatic contralateral approach (in which embolization is performed from the FLR), and the transhepatic ipsilateral approach (in which embolization is performed from the tumor-bearing lobe) are widely used [7]. After PVE, approximately 80–90% of candidates are qualified to undergo hepatectomy, while the remaining patients do not experience adequate FLR hypertrophy [8, 9]. The mean percent FLR hypertrophy was 30.9% with an interval of time 40.3 ± 26.3 days between PVE and curative hepatectomy [9]. The inadequate liver regeneration volume and the presence of tumor progression or metastasis during the long waiting time increase the risk of drop out from the list of subsequent LR. PVE offers an acceptable rate of major complications (less than 5%) including puncture-related complications (vascular injury, biloma, or infection) and embolization-related complications (embolic material migration, non-targeted vein embolization, proximal venous thrombosis, parenchymal infarction, and portal hypertension) [9–11]. Contraindications to PVE in clinical practice consist of portal hypertension, PV thrombus, occlusion of the PV in the FLR, biliary obstruction (biliary drainage before the procedure is required), extrahepatic metastasis, uncorrectable coagulopathy, and renal failure.

2.1.2 Sequential transarterial chemoembolization (TACE) and portal vein embolization (PVE)

Sequential TACE and PVE have been proposed to overcome the aforementioned limitations of PVE alone. The insufficient degree of FLR hypertrophy after PVE alone may be explained by the underlying liver disease that impairs the capacity of liver regeneration, the existence of arterioportal shunt in HCC patients, and the reimbursing rise of hepatic artery (HA) blood flow at the embolized lobe. As shown in a recent systematic review and meta-analysis (SRMA), the sequential TACE and PVE had demonstrated superior advantages in oncological outcomes with greater liver resectability rate and percentage increase in FLR, better overall survival, longer disease-free survival (DFS), as well as its safety with comparable overall morbidity, mortality, and PHLF in compared to PVE alone [12]. In fact, the mean increase in percentage FLR volume varies from 7–18%, according to different studies [13–15]. On the other hand, careful attention must be devoted during glissonean pedicle dissection due to heavy inflammatory adhesion and choledochal varices following the sequential TACE and PVE, which might cause more challenges and difficulties in a subsequent surgery. Another drawback is the risk of severe infarction or necrosis of the residual non-cancerous liver parenchyma, especially in patients with underlying liver disease, due to double occlusion of the arterial and portal venous systems; however, only a mild elevation in liver function test, as well as minimal necrosis in the resected specimen of non-cancerous liver parenchyma were reported in most of the cases [14, 16, 17].

2.1.3 Associated liver partition and portal vein ligation for staged hepatectomy (ALPPS)

The rationale of ALPPS consists of PV ligation on the tumor-bearing lobe and simultaneous severance between the tumor-side liver and the residual liver by liver parenchymal transection during stage one. In stage two, completion of subsequent hepatectomy is achieved by resection of ipsilateral HA, bile duct, and hepatic vein (HV) with a shorter delay of time (usually one or two weeks later). A sufficient FLR volume is ensured by the assessment of computed tomography (CT) or magnetic resonance imaging (MRI)-based liver volumetry measurement. Compared with traditional two-stage hepatectomy (TSH), ALPPS is distinctive with speedy enhancement of adequate FLR hypertrophy following maximal separation of the tumor-bearing lobe to be removed and without risk of dropout due to tumor progression while waiting for liver hypertrophy. As opposed to PVE, data from SRMA have emphasized the advantages of ALPPS with a significant increase in FLR with shorter intervals of time (76% vs. 37%) and a higher rate of stage two completion (100% vs. 77%) [18–20]. Despite preceding benefits, major concerns have been expressed about the safety of ALPPS due to its high rate of morbidity and mortality. The reported major complications range from 21.4% to 54.1% [21–24], and the 90-day mortality rate varies from 5% to 11.8% [22, 25]. Although statistical difference was not reached, ALPPS was proved to have a trend toward higher morbidity and mortality compared to TSH [18, 20]. Thus, in an effort to minimize the invasive complications of this approach, numerous variations on the classical ALPPS have been proposed such as partial ALPPS [26], monosegment ALPPS [27], mini ALPPS [28], radiofrequency ALPPS [29], minimally invasive ALPPS (laparoscopic ALPPS [30] and robotic-assisted ALPPS [31]), tourniquet alPPS [32], hybrid ALPPS [33], salvage ALPPS [34], left and right ALPPS [35]. These modified protocols have ameliorated the safety of ALPPS and improved its morbidity and mortality rate [36]. In terms of oncological outcome, ALPPS offers an overall survival (OS) of 86% at 6 months, falling to 59% at 2 years, and DFS of 59% at 1 year, falling to 41% at 2 years [37]. Indeed, there were no statistical differences regarding OS and DFS between patients who underwent ALPPS and TSH [38].

2.1.4 Liver venous deprivation (LVD)

Another possible approach to achieve the desired FLR volume is LVD, which is associated with simultaneous hepatic vein embolization (HVE) and PVE in the tumor-bearing liver. The concomitant occlusion of the PV and one or even two HV (called extended LVD) induces resonant damage to the ipsilateral lobe and thereby redirects the blood supply to the contralateral lobe, which subsequently accelerates hypertrophy of the FLR. Data from recent SRMA emphasized the promising results of LVD with a significantly higher degree of FLR hypertrophy before major hepatectomy than PVE and with a comparable capacity of regeneration to ALPPS [39]. In addition, LVD was safe, with lower major complications and a 90-day mortality rate compared to PVE and ALPPS [39]. The resection rate following LVD was impressive, with approximately 86–100% of patients who successfully underwent hepatectomy [40–42]. Despite remarkable benefits, the preliminary results of this new technique remain to be carefully explored and validated thoroughly in more studies.

2.2 Anatomic resection (AR) in hepatectomy

2.2.1 The concept of AR

The concept of AR in hepatectomy was initially introduced by the distinguished Japanese professor Makuuchi [43]. AR consists of systematic excision of the tumor-bearing portal tributaries and the corresponding hepatic territory, using PV branches dye-staining method [44] or Glissonean pedicle transection technique [45]. Indeed, the pre-ischemic control of the PV is performed, followed by the complete removal of one or more corresponding Couinaud's segments supplied by a branch of the PV and HA (including segmentectomy, bisectionectomy, trisectionectomy, or hemi-hepatectomy). As liver tumor tends to invade the intrahepatic vascular structure, the entire and thorough elimination of tumor-bearing portal territory suppresses the risk of tumor dissemination (tumor thrombus, daughter nodule, or metastasis) in the corresponding segment through the PV blood flow [46, 47]. Conversely, nonanatomic resection (NAR) is a parenchyma-sparing surgery regardless of the anatomical liver segment, in which the tumor resection is performed with a margin of uninvolved tissue. This protocol is preferred in patients with poor liver function or cirrhosis.

2.2.2 AR versus NAR

Although several retrospective studies did not reveal long-term outcomes advantages of AR vs. NAR [48–51], recently published SRMA have demonstrated the superiority of AR over NAR in terms of OS and DFS [52–54]. However, AR was proven to be associated with longer operation time, significant blood loss, and wider surgical margins [52]. Besides, there was no statistical difference regarding the rate of blood transfusion or postoperative complications between these two techniques [52, 54]. Despite the positive results of the aforementioned SRMA, the divergence benefits of AR vs. NAR might be due to the bias in research design, including diversification in tumor size, tumor location, background of liver function, operation technique, and presence of microvascular invasion (MVI). Therefore, it is currently impossible to reach a final conclusion about the advantages of AR in hepatectomy. Further prospective randomized studies with larger sample size and multicenter design might help to define the true effect of AR.

2.2.3 AR and resection margin (RM) status in the context of MVI

Despite being a matter of controversy, the current data and the clinical practices support the application of AR with curative purposes in reducing the risk of tumor dissemination and metastasis [55, 56]. Previous comprehensive report have focused attention on RM status since micrometastases could expand via invasion of PV branches, which is also known as MVI, even at an early stage with solitary and small tumor [57]. A multi-institutional data with 801 patients revealed the negative impact of RM status and MVI, in which patients with concomitant narrow RM and MVI suffered for postoperative death and recurrence by about two-fold [58]. Given that the incidence of MVI was correspondingly associated with the distance from the primary tumor, a proximal RM and a distal RM of 1 cm are recommended for HCC with a diameter of less than 3 cm, whereas a 1 cm proximal RM and a 2 cm distal RM should be achieved for HCC with diameter higher than 3 cm [57]. Other reports have revealed that the occurrence of PV invasion and intrahepatic micrometastasis was found within 1 cm of the primary tumor, and this phenomenon was rarely broadened to more than 2 cm [57, 59]. An optimal cut-off value of RM higher than 1 cm was then mostly accepted [58, 60, 61]. Given that, it is crucial to apply AR with wide RM, if technically feasible and safe, when the presence of MVI is determined before hepatectomy [58, 61, 62]. A large multicenter propensity score-matched study of 1965 patients highlighted the significance of AR and RM status, in which patients with AR and wide RM group (≥1 cm) had better median OS (78.9 vs. 51.5 vs. 48.0 vs. 36.7 months, $p < 0.001$) and better median recurrence-free survival (RFS) (23.6 vs. 14.8 vs. 17.8 vs. 9.0 months, $P < 0.001$) than those with AR and narrow RM, NAR and wide RM, and NAR and narrow RM groups, respectively [63]. Additionally, regardless of AR or NAR technique, patients with wide RM significantly gained lower operative margin recurrence rates than those with narrow RM [63]. On the other hand, non-tumor-bearing liver parenchyma preservation, also known as parenchyma-sparing LR or NAR, represents a matter of consideration, especially in cirrhotic patients and in patients with insufficient FLR volume. In such a situation when AR and wide RM were unfeasibly obtained at the same time, priority selection should be reserved for AR or for NAR with wide RM? The recent report from 906 HCC patients has emphasized the critical role of wide RM, and this vital feature must be primarily ensured, especially in case of MVI, to improve long-term outcomes [61].

2.3 The minimally invasive liver surgery (MILS)

In 1991, the first case of laparoscopic liver resection (LLR) was incidentally reported in women with benign liver tumor during laparoscopic surgery for gynecologic purposes [64]. Since then, the hepato-biliary-pancreatic (HBP) surgery society has experienced the giant advances of MILS in curative treatment of liver tumors. During the last three decades, the unstoppable developments of the two excellent representatives of MILS, which are LLR and, later, robotic liver resection (RLR), have drastically proved themselves as an alternative approach to traditional open LR. Progress in operational devices, along with accumulated experiences, have promoted the expansion of LLR and RLR indications in clinical practice. The first international consensus conference in Louisville (United States) in 2008 [65], the second meeting in Morioka (Japan) in 2014 [66], and then the recent reunion in Southampton (United Kingdom) in 2017 [67] have witnessed the worldwide adoption of MILS in HBP surgery. Today, LLR should be considered as a standard approach for wedge resection and left lateral or anterior sectionectomy, whereas major hepatectomy, living donor hepatectomy, and ALPPS should be performed at high-volume centers with comprehensive experiences.

Recent SRMA focusing on 13 randomized controlled trials (RCTs) studies in minor LR have emphasized the superiority of LLR over open LR regarding short-term benefits such as lower postoperative complications, lesser blood loss, shorter hospital stay, and faster functional recovery [68]. In terms of long-term oncological outcomes, current evidence encourages LLR with comparable OS and RFS rates compared to open LR [69, 70] or even with better long-term prognosis in cirrhotic HCC patients [71]. On the other hand, the application of RLR in HCC patients seems to overcome LLR in some features such as improvement of surgical manipulations with articulated instruments, better surgical view with three-dimensional (3D) magnified field of vision, greater dexterity and precision with tremor control [72, 73]. As a consequence, RLR approach might be recommended to confer benefits in complex and difficult contexts such as vascular or biliary dissection, suture hemostasis during liver parenchymal dissection, posterosuperior segmentectomy, and biliary-enteric anastomosis [74–76]. Since the implementation of RLR in the field of HBP was recently introduced within 10 years, long-term reports of RLR are scarce. Despite significantly longer surgical time and higher cost, recent SRMA has proved the equivalent benefits of RLR with no statistical difference in length of hospital stay, blood loss, and the incidence of conversion compared to LLR [77]. As there is a lack of robust data, further investigations are required to evaluate and standardize this technique.

2.4 The simulation and navigation in LR

2.4.1 Preoperative simulation using three-dimensional (3D) visualization

Preoperative simulation using 3D imaging software refers to a modality used to virtually reconstruct the liver anatomy by displaying and exploring the intrahepatic structures such as the tumors and the adjacent components. Currently, there are several software which are specified for 3D liver simulation including Synapse Vincent (Fujifilm Medical, Japan), HepaVision (Mevis, Germany) VirtualPlace (AZE, Japan), Ziostation (Ziosoft, Japan), OVA (Hitachi Medical Corporation, Japan), and VR-Render (IRCAD, France) [78]. These tools permit the preoperative design and analysis of the surgical resection plan by investigating the FLR volume and the area perfused by targeted hepatic blood vessels or drained by a specific HV. At initial, CT or MRI imaging data were obtained, stored, and then transferred to the simulation software. Afterward, comprehensive information on the whole liver including hepatic blood vessels (inferior vena cava, HV, HA, and PV), bile duct, liver parenchymal as well as liver tumors were extracted and displayed with marked colors for anatomical identification. According to the patient's status and liver tumor characteristics, different resection planes could be designed to determine the most appropriate approach. The total liver volume and the estimated percent of FLR volume will be automatically analyzed and calculated to avoid the PHLF. In fact, reported data have confirmed the reliability and accuracy of preoperative 3D virtual planning software with a high correlation between the planned and the actual FLR [79, 80].

2.4.2 Intraoperative navigation

The concept of navigation in LR began in 1985 when Professor Makuuchi performed the AR using PV branches dye-staining method; however, this method did not always establish a clear recognition of the segmental boundaries for LR [44, 81]. Since then, various techniques and numerous surgical innovations have been proposed to enhance the safety and precision of LR. In the conventional approach, the adjacent segment was intraoperatively differentiated from each other based on the identification of HV via ultrasonography. In reality, due to the 3D irregular form of each liver segment, the three major HV (left, middle, and right HV) are not sufficient to allow precise AR [82, 83]. In this regard, fluorescent navigation with indocyanine green (ICG), a minimal toxic, cost-effective, and water-soluble fluorescent dye that is rapidly absorbed by the liver and secreted into the bile ducts within minutes after intravenous injection [84], has been comprehensively developed to ameliorate the accuracy in AR, especially in the context of real-time surgery for the last few years. With ICG dying, the shape of the segmental borders including the demarcation line on the liver surface and the subsurface borderline in the liver parenchyma could be clearly identified during liver transection. In the laparoscopic approach, the latest findings in SRMA have supported the application of ICG fluorescent navigation with significantly shorter operation time, intraoperative blood loss, hospital stay, and postoperative complications [85]. It seems that this innovation induced better short-term outcomes, however, its impact on long-term prognosis requires more evidence for the final conclusion.

Another aspect of surgical navigation to take into account is the reflection of the preoperative simulation in the intraoperative field. In reality, the intraoperative demand for real-time visualization of precise liver anatomy is vital to identify the exact segmental landmark in AR and also to assure an R0 resection margin for oncological purposes. To overcome the limitation during the exploration of intraparenchymal structure, the Medical Imaging Projection System (MIPS) was introduced to determine the anatomical landmark during AR, thanks to the combination of ICG emission signal and active projection mapping [86]. This system proved to be more convenient than the conventional fluorescent imaging system in which surgeons, with no requirement of specific goggles, can directly focus on the surgical field without having to move their vision to the displayed screen [86]. In addition, instead of using a handheld camera to operate in the area of interest, the MIPS allows users to perform surgery without physiological tremors and to accommodate liver deformities during surgical manipulation thanks to real-time projection [86]. Besides, the introduction of augmented reality (AR), mixed reality (MR), and 3D navigation technology, an advanced fusion imaging technology that superimposes the 3D virtual images from CT or MRI data onto the liver of a patient, had made an evolution in establishing the exact boundary of LR in real-time with a ratio 1:1 [87]. Its clinical integration into intraoperative procedures has been performed, both in open [88–90] and MILS [91, 92]. The 3D navigation system allows the determination of the exact position of the intraparenchymal targeted lesion [93, 94]. Although current data has revealed some advantages of the aforementioned innovations including increased R0 rate, the elevated number of potential treatable liver lesions, precise AR, improved operation time, and minimized blood loss [95], these technologies require additional evidence for official recognition in the future.

2.5 The utilization of new parenchymal transection devices

In order to complete a successful LR, serious cautions have been reserved for intraoperative hemostatic and biliary control. A meticulous parenchymal dissection are critically required, in which the blood and bile duct system have to be clearly identified. Indeed, the LR procedure consists of two fundamental steps: (1) parenchymal dissection and (2) intrahepatic structures dissection and ligation. Advances in technology with the introduction of new parenchymal transection devices, both in open and MILS approach, have significantly contributed to enhancing this protocol by selectively exposing these structures without damaging them. Since the beginning of hepatectomy with the finger crush technique [96] and then the clamp crushing (CC) technique [97], numerous instruments have been invented and widely used including ultrasonic dissection (such as cavitron ultrasonic surgical aspirator (CUSA) and the harmonic scalpel (HS)), sealing devices (Ligasure), water jet scalpel and vascular stapler.

2.5.1 Ultrasonic dissection

Ultrasonic devices remain one of the most widely used devices in parenchymal transection during LR, especially in donor hepatectomy [98, 99]. The CUSA, the first generation of ultrasonic device, utilizes mechanical wave energy combined with aspiration to fragment and aspirate the liver parenchyma tissue, and then expose biliary ducts over 2 mm and small liver vascular [100]. On the basis of mechanical resistance reflected by the tissue, CUSA induces the fragmentation of hepatocytes without affecting vascular or biliary components since the hepatic parenchyma possesses significantly higher water content and lesser fibrous tissue [101]. This device was helpful and flexible in its use, thanks to its ability to adjust the intensity of dissection according to the degree of liver fibrosis in each patient. Besides individually isolating intrahepatic structures, CUSA offers a well-defined cutting plane as well as precise liver pedicle detection, especially in case of lesions closely located next to the major blood vessels [102]. In the laparoscopic approach, CUSA was useful for the identification of deep-seated intrahepatic vessels [103], especially in the context of challenging parenchyma such as cirrhotic liver [104, 105]. However, as lacking of coagulation function, CUSA's usage requires additional steps with ties, clips, or staplers to complete hemostasis or biliostasis [106].

The harmonic scalpel (HS), an ultrasonic vessel-sealing dissection, mitigated the drawback of the aforementioned device with the capacity of sealing and isolating intrahepatic components up to 3 mm in diameter [107]. This process is achieved using high-frequency ultrasonic energy transmitted between the instrument blades (55,000 Hz) to disrupt the hydrogen bonds and then denature the proteins [108]. Indeed, the hemostasis as well as the biliostasis are completed at low temperature (80°C) with lesser tissue damage as compared to the thermal effect in monopolar electrocautery method [108]. In recipient hepatectomy, HS transection of small HV (lesser than 2 mm) was safer than conventional knot tying without difference in both total procedure and per vessel time [109]. Regarding deep layer parenchymal dissection in LLR, HS was proved to be superior to CUSA in terms of intraoperative blood loss, operation time, and hospital cost, whereas no difference in rate of conversion to laparotomy, length of hospital stay, and postoperative complications was revealed [110]. Findings from recent SRMA have approved the safety of HS in elective parenchymal liver transection with significantly lower overall and major complications [111].

2.5.2 Sealing devices

Sealing devices complete parenchymal transection by sealing small vessels before dissection using a combination of electrothermal energy and pressure to fuse the collagen matrix in the vessel wall [112]. Ligasure, a representative of a sealing device with a bipolar vessel-ligating system, is able to crush the liver parenchyma and simultaneously seal vascular structure up to 7 mm in diameter [112]. In addition, this instrument was designed with a built-in knife that helps to quickly cut the sealed vessel after vascular hemostasis, thereby leading to reduced LR times [113]. In recipient LR during liver transplantation, ligasure was proved to be significantly associated with a shorter hospital stay due to low re-operation rates, postoperative bleeding, and secondary infection related to bleeding in comparison to the conventional monopolar cautery technique [114]. However, despite its safety, findings from RCT revealed no statistical difference in terms of liver transection time, liver transection speed, or the amount of blood loss compared to the CC technique [112]. Further investigations are needed to reach a final conclusion.

2.5.3 Water jet scalpel

The water jet (WJ) technique leverages the high pressure of the fine water flow to cause fragmentation of liver parenchyma, while the exposed elastic intrahepatic structures are individually isolated with spared injury and subsequently ligated [115, 116]. As employed the water flow for breaking liver tissue, the WJ avoids any thermal damage to the remnant liver with significantly lower denaturation thickness in the post LR detached section compared to the conventional CUSA [117]. However, findings from the SRMA of the two RCTs have revealed no statistical difference regarding blood loss, mortality, morbidity, postoperative liver function test, transection time or speed, and median hospital stay between WJ and CUSA [118–120]. The application of the CC technique has even been proven to be quicker than WJ, with a lower rate of blood loss and similar mortality, morbidity, liver dysfunction, and length of hospital stay [118].

2.5.4 Vascular stapler

The technique of vascular stapler (VS) has been described as below: the liver capsule was initially split with diathermy along the transectional landmark, the subsequent transection of liver parenchyma was then crushed stepwise using a vascular clamp and finally dissected with VS [121]. VS has expressed its effectiveness with the capacity to be continually fired in a quick and ready-to-use fashion [113]. An RCT of VS versus CC technique in elective LR has revealed no difference in terms of intra-operative blood loss as well as postoperative morbidity and mortality [122]. Instead, another RCT emphasized the superiority of VS over ligasure with significantly lesser blood loss and shorter operation time, whereas the surgical morbidity and the grade of complication were comparable [123].

2.6 Liver transplantation (LT) versus LR

In cirrhotic HCC patients with worse liver function, LT represents an ideal alternative for curative purposes to LR, in which both the existing tumor and the preneoplastic underlying liver parenchyma are treated. Given the shortage of donor organs along with the huge number of patients on the waiting list, LT becomes less eligible for a certain amount of patients. In addition, such challenges impede the wide adoption of LT including the heavy financial requirement owing to the high cost of transplant operation and long-term use of immunosuppressant (IS), the availability of a specialized and skilled surgical team as well as the adherence to the side effects arising from lifelong IS use. Thus, the selection between these two curative surgical approaches remains a topic of passionate debate. LR seems to be a preferred therapy for HCC patients with reserved liver function, whereas LT is an appropriate option in case of impaired liver function. Besides, concerns about the long-term outcomes of HCC for LR versus LT have recently gained much attention. Despite longer hospital stay, LT has provided greater overall and event-free survival rates with comparable morbidity and mortality rates than LR [124]. The surveillance, epidemiology, and end results program (SEER) database, which generally represents the entire US population, has also revealed that patients with LT offered a lower risk of overall mortality and cancer-free mortality than those with LR [125]. Likewise, the latest findings from SRMA and from meta-analysis of meta-analyses have again emphasized the superiority of LT over LR with regard to long-term outcomes [111, 126]. Indeed, data from 63 studies involving 8178 cases of LT and 11,626 cases of LR have concluded that LT provided better 5 years OS and RFS compared to LR but not in short-term intervals [111, 126]. As regards to recurrence, current evidence supports the superior role of salvage LT, in which initial LR with curative purpose was performed and followed by LT due to tumor recurrence, then repeat LR with better disease-specific and RFS for treating transplantation-eligible patients with intrahepatic HCC recurrence, even in Child-Pugh class A cirrhotic patients [127].

3. Conclusion

LR remains the cornerstone of HCC treatment in terms of safety, feasibility, and effectiveness. LT represents an optimal alternative to LR in case of severely impaired liver function. Recent inventions and innovations have significantly contributed to the preoperative, intraoperative, and postoperative management of HCC patients. Such attempts have been made to reduce blood loss and improve oncological outcomes. With a deeper understanding of segmental liver anatomy, assistance from simulation and navigation systems, advances in FLR optimization, MILS, new parenchymal transection devices, and LT, liver surgeons should tailor the surgical plan according to each individual to achieve the best outcome for patients.

Conflict of interest

The authors declare no conflict of interest.

Nomenclature

3D	three-dimensional
ALPPS	associated liver partition and portal vein ligation for staged hepatectomy
AR	augmented reality
AR	anatomic resection
CC	clamp crushing
CT	computed tomography
CUSA	cavitron ultrasonic surgical aspirator
DFS	disease-free survival
HA	hepatic artery
HBP	hepato-biliary-pancreatic
HCC	hepatocellular carcinoma
HS	harmonic scalpel
HV	hepatic vein
HVE	hepatic vein embolization
FLR	future liver remnant
ICG	indocyanine green
IS	immunosuppressant
LLR	laparoscopic liver resection
LR	liver resection
LVD	liver venous deprivation
LT	liver transplantation
LTA	local tumor ablation
MILS	minimally invasive liver surgery
MIPS	medical imaging projection system
MR	mixed reality
MRI	magnetic resonance imaging
MVI	microvascular invasion
NAR	nonanatomic resection
PHLF	post-hepatectomy liver failure
PV	portal vein
PVE	portal vein embolization
RCT	randomized controlled trial
RFS	recurrence-free survival
RLR	robotic liver resection
RM	resection margin
SRMA	systematic review and meta-analysis

TACE	transarterial chemoembolization
TSH	two-stage hepatectomy
TLV	total liver volume
VS	vascular stapler
WJ	water jet

Author details

Nguyen Hai Nam[1,2]

1 Department of Liver Tumor, Cancer Center, Cho Ray Hospital, Ho Chi Minh City, Vietnam

2 Liver Transplant Unit, Cancer Center, Cho Ray Hospital, Ho Chi Minh City, Vietnam

*Address all correspondence to: dr.nguyenhainam@gmail.com

References

[1] Bray F et al. Global cancer statistics 2018: GLOBOCAN estimates of incidence and mortality worldwide for 36 cancers in 185 countries. CA: a Cancer Journal for Clinicians. 2018;**68**(6):394-424

[2] Sung H et al. Global cancer statistics 2020: GLOBOCAN estimates of incidence and mortality worldwide for 36 cancers in 185 countries. CA: a Cancer Journal for Clinicians. 2021;**71**(3):209-249

[3] Galle PR et al. EASL clinical practice guidelines: Management of hepatocellular carcinoma. Journal of Hepatology. 2018;**69**(1):182-236

[4] Guglielmi A et al. How much remnant is enough in liver resection? Digestive Surgery. 2012;**29**(1):6-17

[5] Abdalla EK et al. Improving Resectability of Hepatic colorectal metastases: Expert consensus statement. Annals of Surgical Oncology. 2006;**13**(10):1271-1280

[6] Makuuchi M et al. Preoperative portal embolization to increase safety of major hepatectomy for hilar bile duct carcinoma: A preliminary report. Surgery. 1990;**107**(5):521-527

[7] Avritscher R et al. Percutaneous transhepatic portal vein embolization: Rationale, technique, and outcomes. Seminars in Interventional Radiology. 2008;**25**(2):132-145

[8] Cassese G et al. Portal vein embolization failure: Current strategies and future perspectives to improve liver hypertrophy before major oncological liver resection. World Journal of Gastrointestinal Oncology. 2022;**14**(11):2088-2096

[9] Charalel RA et al. Systematic reviews and meta-analyses of portal vein embolization, associated liver partition and portal vein ligation, and radiation lobectomy outcomes in hepatocellular carcinoma patients. Current Oncology Reports. 2021;**23**(11):135

[10] van Lienden KP et al. Portal vein embolization before liver resection: A systematic review. Cardio Vascular and Interventional Radiology. 2013;**36**(1):25-34

[11] Yeom YK, Shin JH. Complications of portal vein embolization: Evaluation on cross-sectional imaging. Korean Journal of Radiology. 2015;**16**(5):1079-1085

[12] Liao Y et al. Sequential transcatheter arterial chemoembolization and portal vein embolization before hepatectomy for the management of patients with hepatocellular carcinoma: A systematic review and meta-analysis. Updates in Surgery. 2023;**75**(7):1741-1750

[13] Ogata S et al. Sequential arterial and portal vein embolizations before right hepatectomy in patients with cirrhosis and hepatocellular carcinoma. The British Journal of Surgery. 2006;**93**(9):1091-1098

[14] Park GC et al. Sequential transcatheter arterial chemoembolization and portal vein embolization before right hemihepatectomy in patients with hepatocellular carcinoma. Hepatobiliary & Pancreatic Diseases International. 2020;**19**(3):244-251

[15] Yoo H et al. Sequential transcatheter arterial chemoembolization and portal vein embolization versus portal vein embolization only before major hepatectomy for patients with

hepatocellular carcinoma. Annals of Surgical Oncology. 2011;**18**(5):1251-1257

[16] Zhang CW et al. Simultaneous transcatheter arterial chemoembolization and portal vein embolization for patients with large hepatocellular carcinoma before major hepatectomy. World Journal of Gastroenterology. 2020;**26**(30):4489-4500

[17] Aoki T et al. Sequential preoperative arterial and portal venous embolizations in patients with hepatocellular carcinoma. Archives of Surgery. 2004;**139**(7):766-774

[18] Liu Y et al. A systematic review and meta-analysis of associating liver partition and portal vein ligation for staged hepatectomy (ALPPS) versus traditional staged hepatectomy. Medicine (Baltimore). 2019;**98**(15):e15229

[19] Zhou Z et al. Associating liver partition and portal vein ligation for staged hepatectomy versus conventional two-stage hepatectomy: A systematic review and meta-analysis. World Journal of Surgical Oncology. 2017;**15**(1):227

[20] Eshmuminov D et al. Meta-analysis of associating liver partition with portal vein ligation and portal vein occlusion for two-stage hepatectomy. The British Journal of Surgery. 2016;**103**(13):1768-1782

[21] Li PP et al. Associating liver partition and portal vein ligation for staged hepatectomy versus sequential transarterial chemoembolization and portal vein embolization in staged hepatectomy for HBV-related hepatocellular carcinoma: A randomized comparative study. Hepatobiliary Surgery and Nutrition. 2022;**11**(1):38-51

[22] Maupoey Ibáñez J et al. From conventional two-stage hepatectomy to ALPPS: Fifteen years of experience in a hepatobiliary surgery unit. Hepatobiliary & Pancreatic Diseases International. 2021;**20**(6):542-550

[23] Serenari M et al. Minimally invasive stage 1 to protect against the risk of liver failure: Results from the hepatocellular carcinoma series of the associating liver partition and portal vein ligation for staged hepatectomy Italian registry. Journal of Laparoendoscopic & Advanced Surgical Techniques. Part A. 2020;**30**(10):1082-1089

[24] Zhang J et al. Application of associating liver partition and portal vein ligation for staged hepatectomy for hepatocellular carcinoma related to hepatitis B virus: Comparison with traditional one-stage right hepatectomy. Translational Cancer Research. 2020;**9**(9):5371-5379

[25] Petrowsky H et al. First long-term oncologic results of the ALPPS procedure in a large cohort of patients with colorectal liver metastases. Annals of Surgery. 2020;**272**(5):793-800

[26] Petrowsky H et al. Is partial-ALPPS safer than ALPPS? A single-center experience. Annals of Surgery. 2015;**261**(4):e90-e92

[27] Schadde E et al. Monosegment ALPPS hepatectomy: Extending resectability by rapid hypertrophy. Surgery. 2015;**157**(4):676-689

[28] de Santibañes E et al. Inverting the ALPPS paradigm by minimizing first stage impact: The mini-ALPPS technique. Langenbeck's Archives of Surgery. 2016;**401**(4):557-563

[29] Rong Z, Lu Q, Yan J. Totally laparoscopic radiofrequency-assisted liver partition with portal vein ligation for hepatocellular carcinoma in

cirrhotic liver. Medicine (Baltimore). 2017;**96**(51):e9432

[30] Xiao L, Li JW, Zheng SG. Totally laparoscopic ALPPS in the treatment of cirrhotic hepatocellular carcinoma. Surgical Endoscopy. 2015;**29**(9):2800-2801

[31] Vicente E et al. First ALPPS procedure using a total robotic approach. Surgical Oncology. 2016;**25**(4):457

[32] Robles R et al. Tourniquet modification of the associating liver partition and portal ligation for staged hepatectomy procedure. The British Journal of Surgery. 2014;**101**(9):1129-1134 discussion 1134

[33] Li J et al. Avoid "all-touch" by hybrid ALPPS to achieve oncological efficacy. Annals of Surgery. 2016;**263**(1):e6-e7

[34] Tschuor C et al. Salvage parenchymal liver transection for patients with insufficient volume increase after portal vein occlusion -- an extension of the ALPPS approach. European Journal of Surgical Oncology. 2013;**39**(11):1230-1235

[35] Gauzolino R et al. The ALPPS technique for bilateral colorectal metastases: Three "variations on a theme". Updates in Surgery. 2013;**65**(2):141-148

[36] Chan KS, Low JK, Shelat VG. Associated liver partition and portal vein ligation for staged hepatectomy: A review. Translational Gastroenterology and Hepatology. 2020;**5**:37

[37] Schadde E et al. Early survival and safety of ALPPS: First report of the international ALPPS registry. Annals of Surgery. 2014;**260**(5):829-836; discussion 836-8

[38] Díaz Vico T et al. Two stage hepatectomy (TSH) versus ALPPS for initially unresectable colorectal liver metastases: A systematic review and meta-analysis. European Journal of Surgical Oncology. 2023;**49**(3):550-559

[39] Gavriilidis P et al. Simultaneous portal and hepatic vein embolization is better than portal embolization or ALPPS for hypertrophy of future liver remnant before major hepatectomy: A systematic review and network meta-analysis. Hepatobiliary & Pancreatic Diseases International. 2023;**22**(3):221-227

[40] Guiu B et al. Simultaneous trans-hepatic portal and hepatic vein embolization before major hepatectomy: The liver venous deprivation technique. European Radiology. 2016;**26**(12):4259-4267

[41] Cassese G et al. Liver venous deprivation versus associating liver partition and portal vein ligation for staged hepatectomy for Colo-rectal liver metastases: A comparison of early and late kinetic growth rates, and perioperative and oncological outcomes. Surgical Oncology. 2022;**43**:101812

[42] Cassese G et al. Liver venous deprivation versus portal vein embolization before major hepatectomy for colorectal liver metastases: A retrospective comparison of short- and medium-term outcomes. Journal of Gastrointestinal Surgery. 2023;**27**(2):296-305

[43] Makuuchi M et al. Safety of hemihepatic vascular occlusion during resection of the liver. Surgery, Gynecology & Obstetrics. 1987;**164**(2):155-158

[44] Makuuchi M, Hasegawa H, Yamazaki S. Ultrasonically guided subsegmentectomy. Surgery, Gynecology & Obstetrics. 1985;**161**(4):346-350

[45] Takasaki K. Glissonean pedicle transection method for hepatic resection: A new concept of liver segmentation. Journal of Hepato-Biliary-Pancreatic Surgery. 1998;**5**(3):286-291

[46] Huber AR et al. Accuracy of vascular invasion reporting in hepatocellular carcinoma before and after implementation of subspecialty surgical pathology sign-out. Indian Journal of Pathology & Microbiology. 2017;**60**(4):501-504

[47] Kang KJ, Ahn KS. Anatomical resection of hepatocellular carcinoma: A critical review of the procedure and its benefits on survival. World Journal of Gastroenterology. 2017;**23**(7):1139-1146

[48] Marubashi S et al. Analysis of recurrence patterns after anatomical or non-anatomical resection for hepatocellular carcinoma. Annals of Surgical Oncology. 2015;**22**(7):2243-2252

[49] Okamura Y et al. Anatomic versus nonanatomic hepatectomy for a solitary hepatocellular carcinoma: A case-controlled study with propensity score matching. Journal of Gastrointestinal Surgery. 2014;**18**(11):1994-2002

[50] Marubashi S et al. Anatomical versus non-anatomical resection for hepatocellular carcinoma. The British Journal of Surgery. 2015;**102**(7):776-784

[51] Tomimaru Y et al. Equivalent outcomes after anatomical and non-anatomical resection of small hepatocellular carcinoma in patients with preserved liver function. Digestive Diseases and Sciences. 2012;**57**(7):1942-1948

[52] Liu H et al. Anatomical vs nonanatomical liver resection for solitary hepatocellular carcinoma: A systematic review and meta-analysis. World Journal of Gastrointestinal Oncology. 2021;**13**(11):1833-1846

[53] Dai XM et al. Oncological outcomes of anatomic versus non-anatomic resections for small hepatocellular carcinoma: Systematic review and meta-analysis of propensity-score matched studies. World Journal of Surgical Oncology. 2022;**20**(1):299

[54] Shin SW et al. Effect of anatomical liver resection for hepatocellular carcinoma: A systematic review and meta-analysis. International Journal of Surgery. 2023;**109**(9):2784-2793

[55] Shimizu A et al. Impact of anatomical liver resection for hepatocellular carcinoma in preventing early-phase local recurrence after surgery. Journal of Hepato-Biliary-Pancreatic Sciences. 2024:1-15

[56] Shindoh J et al. Successful anatomic resection of tumor-bearing portal territory delays long-term stage progression of hepatocellular carcinoma. Annals of Surgical Oncology. 2021;**28**(2):844-853

[57] Shi M et al. Micrometastases of solitary hepatocellular carcinoma and appropriate resection margin. World Journal of Surgery. 2004;**28**(4):376-381

[58] Han J et al. The impact of resection margin and microvascular invasion on long-term prognosis after curative resection of hepatocellular carcinoma: A multi-institutional study. HPB: The Official Journal of the International Hepato Pancreato Biliary Association. 2019;**21**(8):962-971

[59] Nakashima Y et al. Portal vein invasion and intrahepatic micrometastasis in small hepatocellular carcinoma by gross type. Hepatology Research. 2003;**26**(2):142-147

[60] Shi M et al. Partial hepatectomy with wide versus narrow resection margin for solitary hepatocellular carcinoma: A prospective randomized trial. Annals of Surgery. 2007;**245**(1):36-43

[61] Liu J et al. The comparison of surgical margins and type of Hepatic resection for hepatocellular carcinoma with microvascular invasion. The Oncologist. 2023;**28**(11):e1043-e1051

[62] Shi C et al. Anatomic resection and wide resection margin play an important role in hepatectomy for hepatocellular carcinoma with peritumoural micrometastasis. ANZ Journal of Surgery. 2019;**89**(11):E482-e486

[63] Zhang XP et al. Significance of anatomical resection and resection margin status in patients with HBV-related hepatocellular carcinoma and microvascular invasion: A multicenter propensity score-matched study. International Journal of Surgery. 2023;**109**(4):679-688

[64] Reich H et al. Laparoscopic excision of benign liver lesions. Obstetrics and Gynecology. 1991; **78**(5 Pt 2):956-958

[65] Buell JF et al. The international position on laparoscopic liver surgery: The Louisville statement, 2008. Annals of Surgery. 2009;**250**(5):825-830

[66] Wakabayashi G et al. Recommendations for laparoscopic liver resection: A report from the second international consensus conference held in Morioka. Annals of Surgery. 2015;**261**(4):619-629

[67] Abu Hilal M et al. The Southampton consensus guidelines for laparoscopic liver surgery: From indication to implementation. Annals of Surgery. Jul 2018;**268**(1):11-18

[68] Haney CM et al. A systematic review and meta-analysis of randomized controlled trials comparing laparoscopic and open liver resection. HPB: The Official Journal of the International Hepato Pancreato Biliary Association. 2021;**23**(10):1467-1481

[69] Wang ZY et al. Laparoscopic versus open major liver resection for hepatocellular carcinoma: Systematic review and meta-analysis of comparative cohort studies. BMC Cancer. 2019;**19**(1):1047

[70] Ciria R et al. A systematic review and meta-analysis comparing the short- and long-term outcomes for laparoscopic and open liver resections for hepatocellular carcinoma: Updated results from the European guidelines meeting on laparoscopic liver Surgery, Southampton, UK, 2017. Annals of Surgical Oncology. 2019;**26**(1):252-263

[71] Jiang S et al. Laparoscopic versus open hepatectomy in short- and long-term outcomes of the hepatocellular carcinoma patients with cirrhosis: A systematic review and meta-analysis. Journal of Laparoendoscopic & Advanced Surgical Techniques. Part A. 2019;**29**(5):643-654

[72] Ho CM et al. Systematic review of robotic liver resection. Surgical Endoscopy. 2013;**27**(3):732-739

[73] Dalsgaard T et al. Robotic Surgery is less physically demanding than laparoscopic Surgery: Paired cross sectional study. Annals of Surgery. 2020;**271**(1):106-113

[74] Kato Y, Sugioka A, Uyama I. Robotic liver resection for liver malignancy. Gan to Kagaku Ryoho. 2023;**50**(4):437-441

[75] Zhao Z et al. Robotic hepatic resection in postero-superior

region of liver. Updates in Surgery. 2021;**73**(3):1007-1014

[76] Goodsell KE, Park JO. Robotic hepatectomy: Current evidence and future directions. Minerva Surgery. 2023;**78**(5):525-536

[77] Aboudou T et al. Laparoscopic versus robotic hepatectomy: A systematic review and meta-analysis. Journal of Clinical Medicine. 2022;**11**(19):5831

[78] Mise Y et al. Virtual liver resection: Computer-assisted operation planning using a three-dimensional liver representation. Journal of Hepato-Biliary-Pancreatic Sciences. 2013;**20**(2):157-164

[79] Simpson AL et al. Liver planning software accurately predicts postoperative liver volume and measures early regeneration. Journal of the American College of Surgeons. 2014;**219**(2):199-207

[80] Bégin A et al. Accuracy of preoperative automatic measurement of the liver volume by CT-scan combined to a 3D virtual surgical planning software (3DVSP). Surgical Endoscopy. 2014;**28**(12):3408-3412

[81] Allaire M et al. New frontiers in liver resection for hepatocellular carcinoma. JHEP Reports. 2020;**2**(4):100134

[82] Wakabayashi T et al. Landmarks to identify segmental borders of the liver: A review prepared for PAM-HBP expert consensus meeting 2021. Journal of Hepato-Biliary-Pancreatic Sciences. 2022;**29**(1):82-98

[83] Nishino H et al. What is a precise anatomic resection of the liver? Proposal of a new evaluation method in the era of fluorescence navigation surgery. Journal of Hepato-Biliary-Pancreatic Sciences. 2021;**28**(6):479-488

[84] Reinhart MB et al. Indocyanine green: Historical context, current applications, and future considerations. Surgical Innovation. 2016;**23**(2):166-175

[85] Liu Y et al. Meta-analysis of indocyanine green fluorescence imaging-guided laparoscopic hepatectomy. Photodiagnosis and Photodynamic Therapy. 2021;**35**:102354

[86] Nishino H et al. Real-time navigation for liver Surgery using projection mapping with Indocyanine green fluorescence: Development of the novel medical imaging projection system. Annals of Surgery. 2018;**267**(6):1134-1140

[87] Miyata A et al. Simulation and navigation liver surgery: An update after 2,000 virtual hepatectomies. Global Health & Medicine. 2020;**2**(5):298-305

[88] Tang R et al. Augmented reality navigation in open surgery for hilar cholangiocarcinoma resection with hemihepatectomy using video-based in situ three-dimensional anatomical modeling: A case report. Medicine. 2017;**96**(37):e8083

[89] Saito Y et al. Intraoperative 3D hologram support with mixed reality techniques in liver Surgery. Annals of Surgery. 2020;**271**(1):e4-e7

[90] Yasuda J et al. Novel navigation system by augmented reality technology using a tablet PC for hepatobiliary and pancreatic surgery. The International Journal of Medical Robotics and Computer Assisted Surgery. 2018;**14**(5):e1921

[91] Pessaux P et al. Towards cybernetic surgery: Robotic and augmented reality-assisted liver segmentectomy. Langenbeck's Archives of Surgery. 2015;**400**(3):381-385

[92] Schneider C et al. Comparison of manual and semi-automatic registration in augmented reality image-guided liver surgery: A clinical feasibility study. Surgical Endoscopy. 2020;**34**(10):4702-4711

[93] Pelanis E et al. Evaluation of a novel navigation platform for laparoscopic liver surgery with organ deformation compensation using injected fiducials. Medical Image Analysis. 2021;**69**:101946

[94] Thomas MN et al. Navigated laparoscopic microwave ablation of tumour mimics in pig livers: A randomized ex-vivo experimental trial. Surgical Endoscopy. 2021;**35**(12):6763-6769

[95] Wahba R et al. Clinical use of augmented reality, mixed reality, three-dimensional-navigation and artificial intelligence in liver surgery. Artificial Intelligence in Gastroenterology. 2021;**2**:94-104

[96] Gans H et al. Evaluation of the effects of the finger fracture technique used in hepatic resection. Surgery, Gynecology & Obstetrics. 1974;**138**(6):885-890

[97] Ishizaki Y et al. Hepatectomy using traditional Péan clamp-crushing technique under intermittent Pringle maneuver. American Journal of Surgery. 2008;**196**(3):353-357

[98] Han JR et al. How to use energy device for pure laparoscopic donor hepatectomy. Laparoscopic Surgery. 2020;**4**:38

[99] Cho JY et al. Survey results of the expert meeting on laparoscopic living donor hepatectomy and literature review. Digestive Surgery. 2018;**35**(4):289-293

[100] Poon RT. Current techniques of liver transection. HPB: The Official Journal of the International Hepato Pancreato Biliary Association. 2007;**9**(3):166-173

[101] Huang KW et al. Impact of cavitron ultrasonic surgical aspirator (CUSA) and bipolar radiofrequency device (Habib-4X) based hepatectomy for hepatocellular carcinoma on tumour recurrence and disease-free survival. Oncotarget. 2017;**8**(55):93644-93654

[102] Fernando B et al. Main instruments for hepatic transection and minimally invasive pedicle dissection. In: Glissonean Pedicles Approach in Minimally Invasive Liver Surgery. 2023. pp. 29-38. Available from: https://link.springer.com/chapter/10.1007/978-3-031-35295-9_4

[103] Ho CM et al. Total laparoscopic limited anatomical resection for centrally located hepatocellular carcinoma in cirrhotic liver. Surgical Endoscopy. 2013;**27**(5):1820-1825

[104] Cheung TT et al. Pure laparoscopic hepatectomy versus open hepatectomy for hepatocellular carcinoma in 110 patients with liver cirrhosis: A propensity analysis at a single Center. Annals of Surgery. 2016;**264**(4):612-620

[105] Yoon YI et al. Pure laparoscopic versus open right hepatectomy for hepatocellular carcinoma in patients with cirrhosis: A propensity score matched analysis. Annals of Surgery. 2017;**265**(5):856-863

[106] Fabrizio R et al. In: Hepatic Surgery A, Hesham, editors. The Aim of Technology during Liver Resection — A Strategy to Minimize Blood Loss during Liver Surgery. IntechOpen: Rijeka; 2013. p. Ch. 7

[107] McCarus SD, Parnell LKS. The origin and evolution of the HARMONIC® scalpel. Surgical Technology International. 2019;**35**:201-213

[108] Siperstein AE, Berber E, Morkoyun E. The use of the harmonic

scalpel vs conventional knot tying for vessel ligation in thyroid Surgery. Archives of Surgery. 2002;**137**(2):137-142

[109] Olmez A et al. Comparison of harmonic scalpel versus conventional knot tying for transection of short hepatic veins at liver transplantation: Prospective randomized study. Transplantation Proceedings. 2012;**44**(6):1717-1719

[110] Yang Y et al. Laparoscopic liver resection with "ultrasonic scalpel mimic CUSA" technique. Surgical Endoscopy. 2022;**36**(12):8927-8934

[111] Kamarajah SK et al. A systematic review and network meta-analysis of parenchymal transection techniques during hepatectomy: An appraisal of current randomised controlled trials. HPB: The Official Journal of the International Hepato Pancreato Biliary Association. 2020;**22**(2):204-214

[112] Ikeda M et al. The vessel sealing system (LigaSure) in hepatic resection: A randomized controlled trial. Annals of Surgery. 2009;**250**(2):199-203

[113] Aragon RJ, Solomon NL. Techniques of hepatic resection. Journal of Gastrointestinal Oncology. 2012;**3**(1):28-40

[114] Lee JM et al. LigaSure versus monopolar cautery for recipient hepatectomy in liver transplantation: A propensity score-matched analysis. Annals of Translational Medicine. 2021;**9**(13):1050

[115] Rau HG, Duessel AP, Wurzbacher S. The use of water-jet dissection in open and laparoscopic liver resection. HPB: The Official Journal of the International Hepato Pancreato Biliary Association. 2008;**10**(4):275-280

[116] Une Y et al. Liver resection using a water jet. Cancer Chemotherapy and Pharmacology. 1989;**23**(Suppl):S74-S77

[117] Hanaki T et al. Influence of the water jet system vs cavitron ultrasonic surgical aspirator for liver resection on the remnant liver. World Journal of Clinical Cases. 2022;**10**(20):6855-6864

[118] Pamecha V et al. Techniques for liver parenchymal transection: A meta-analysis of randomized controlled trials. HPB: The Official Journal of the International Hepato Pancreato Biliary Association. 2009;**11**(4):275-281

[119] Rau HG et al. Surgical techniques in hepatic resections: Ultrasonic aspirator versus jet-cutter. A prospective randomized clinical trial. Zentralblatt für Chirurgie. 2001;**126**(8):586-590

[120] Lesurtel M et al. How should transection of the liver be performed?: A prospective randomized study in 100 consecutive patients: Comparing four different transection strategies. Annals of Surgery. 2005;**242**(6):814-822, discussion 822-3

[121] Schemmer P et al. Stapler hepatectomy is a safe dissection technique: Analysis of 300 patients. World Journal of Surgery. 2006;**30**(3):419-430

[122] Rahbari NN et al. Randomized clinical trial of stapler versus clamp-crushing transection in elective liver resection. The British Journal of Surgery. 2014;**101**(3):200-207

[123] Fritzmann J et al. Randomized clinical trial of stapler hepatectomy versus LigaSure™ transection in elective hepatic resection. The British Journal of Surgery. 2018;**105**(9):1119-1127

[124] Aksoy SO et al. Comparison of resection and liver transplant

in treatment of hepatocellular carcinoma. Experimental and Clinical Transplantation. 2020;**18**(6):712-718

[125] Zhang K et al. Survival outcomes of liver transplantation versus liver resection among patients with hepatocellular carcinoma: A SEER-based longitudinal study. Journal of the Formosan Medical Association. 2019;**118**(4):790-796

[126] Martinino A et al. Liver transplantation vs liver resection in HCC: Promoting extensive collaborative research through a survival meta-analysis of meta-analyses. Frontiers in Oncology. 2024;**14**:1366607

[127] Yoon Y-I et al. Salvage living donor liver transplantation versus repeat liver resection for patients with recurrent hepatocellular carcinoma and child-Pugh class a liver cirrhosis: A propensity score-matched comparison. American Journal of Transplantation. 2022;**22**(1):165-176

Chapter 8

The Role of Radiation in the Treatment of Hepatocellular Carcinoma

Christian N. Schill and William H. Smith

Abstract

In the past two decades, Radiation Therapy (RT) has become a cornerstone in the treatment of hepatocellular carcinoma (HCC), thanks to significant advancements in radiation delivery techniques. Previously, conventional RT played a limited role in treating HCC due to the high risk of toxicity to normal liver tissue. However, with the introduction of advanced techniques like stereotactic body radiation (SBRT), radiation has become more precise and targeted. SBRT, in particular, has emerged as a valuable locoregional therapy for HCC patients who are not candidates for surgery or other local treatments. This chapter aims to explore the evolving role of RT in multidisciplinary HCC care and highlight the technique, indications, and supporting literature for SBRT and proton therapy in early and intermediate HCC treatment. Additionally, we will delve into the palliative uses of RT for pain relief and tumor burden reduction in HCC patients. Finally, we will review recent advances in RT, such as adaptive radiotherapy and biological-guided radiotherapy, discussing their potential impact on HCC treatment.

Keywords: hepatocellular carcinoma, stereotactic body radiation therapy, biology-guided radiotherapy, adaptive radiotherapy, radiotherapy, palliative radiation therapy

1. Introduction

Crouched over a wooden table scattered with handwritten parchments, glass tubes, and metal coils in a dimly lit lab at the University of Würzburg, a German Scientist named Wilhelm Conrad Röntgen would accidentally discover the beams we would come to know now as X-rays. He would shut himself away in that lab for months, consumed by the mystery of these invisible rays, conducting a series of experiments to understand their nature and properties. His experiments would even include exposing his own wife's hand to the beams in front of a film, which revealed the bones and structures within, marking a pivotal moment in the history of modern medicine (**Figure 1**).

Röntgen's groundbreaking discovery was met with immediate interest and excitement from the scientific community. Just 3 days after his report on these

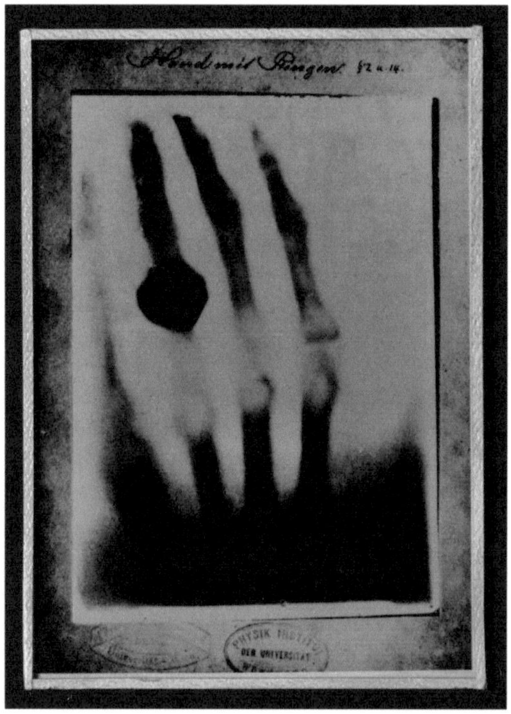

Figure 1.
The first X-ray ever taken of the hand of Anna Bertha Ludwig, the wife of Röntgen. She would famously exclaim upon looking at the X-ray: "I have seen my death!".

experiments was published in January of 1896, a woman with an ulcerating breast cancer would become the first recorded patient treated with radiation. This marked the beginning of a new era in cancer treatment, as physicians began to explore the therapeutic potential of X-rays in targeting and destroying cancerous cells.

Since then, X-rays have been applied to the treatment of benign and malignant tumors arising from every organ in the body. In the field of radiation oncology, X-ray-based therapies have evolved significantly, with the development of techniques such as intensity-modulated radiation therapy (IMRT), stereotactic body radiation therapy (SBRT), and proton therapy, among others. Today, radiation therapy is one of the three key pillars of modern cancer treatment, alongside systemic drug therapies and surgery. Radiation oncology has become a subspecialty field of medicine, with highly trained clinicians prescribing, planning, and delivering highly conformal treatment to a plethora of cancers. For many tumors, radiation therapy (RT) has become a key part of the standard of care, such as in the adjuvant setting in breast cancer or in combination with hormonal therapy in high-risk prostate cancer. In the case of hepatocellular carcinoma (HCC), RT has emerged as an important treatment modality among nonoperative candidates, particularly with the advent of SBRT.

This chapter reviews the specific role that radiation therapy plays in the care of patients with HCC. It focuses on the current approach to HCC radiation therapy, namely, SBRT or proton therapy, and discusses recent advances that may shape the future of HCC treatment in the coming decades.

2. The role of radiation in the multidisciplinary treatment of cancer

As evident in this textbook, cancer treatment is typically multifaceted, necessitating input and collaboration from various physician specialists. RT is a pivotal component forming the third pillar in the essential triangle of cancer care, also including chemotherapy and surgery. RT employs high-energy photons directed at solid tumors to bolster locoregional control, inhibit the spread of primary tumors, prevent metastases, extend survival, and alleviate tumor-associated pain and discomfort. In this section, we will delve into the principles of radiobiology that underlie the use of RT and elaborate on some of its applications in clinical cancer care.

2.1 Rationale for treating solid tumors with ionizing radiation

To understand the role of RT in cancer care, it is important to first understand the mechanisms by which RT exerts its anticancer effects. Radiation itself can represent any form of high energy moving subatomic particles, whether this be high-energy photons, electrons, or protons. These can be given off by radioactive decay of elements such as radium or uranium, or, as is seen more often clinically, high-energy particles can be produced through the use of linear accelerators (LinAcs). LinAcs are capable of producing ionizing radiation by shooting high-energy electrons at high speeds onto an elemental target, such as tungsten, causing the production of high-energy photons *via* Bremstrahlung radiation, which are then directed at the tumor.

There are various forms of radiation present in our modern world, such as the waves utilized to enable the connectivity of our cellphones. However, such radiation is generally not harmful to human cells because it lacks sufficient energy to ionize atoms. High-energy radiation utilized in clinical oncology, on the other hand, possesses the capability to ionize atoms by removing valence orbital electrons, leaving behind charged radicals that are highly reactive with nearby atoms [1]. This ionizing energy can exert both direct and indirect effects on the DNA of exposed cells. Direct effects occur when atoms in the DNA of cells are directly ionized, whereas indirect effects stem from the generation of free hydroxide radicals that subsequently damage the nucleic acids of the cell [2]. **Figure 2** illustrates the difference between direct and indirect DNA damage. Although both types of damage contribute to the clinical effects of radiation, indirect DNA damage typically prevails as the primary mechanism inducing cellular damage following radiation exposure [1].

When interacting with DNA, hydroxide radicals have the potential to cause double-stranded DNA breaks, a severe form of damage that can induce cell death if present during the division process through a process called mitotic catastrophe [3]. Given the severe implication of double-strand DNA breaks, normal cells have numerous and redundant mechanisms to repair such damage including nonhomologous end joining or homologous recombination [3]. Malignant cells, in contrast, have typically undergone numerous mutations to circumvent cell cycle checkpoint controls, often leading to the loss of DNA repair mechanisms. While this benefits highly replicating tumors seeking to acquire more mutations for invasive and metastatic potential, it also means that the burden of DNA damage is significantly higher when exposed to DNA insults including radiation [3]. Therefore, chemotherapy and radiation therapy target DNA because they preferentially impact tumor cells. Conversely, normal cells in the body typically retain intact DNA repair mechanisms, enabling them to effectively repair DNA damage secondary to radiation exposure.

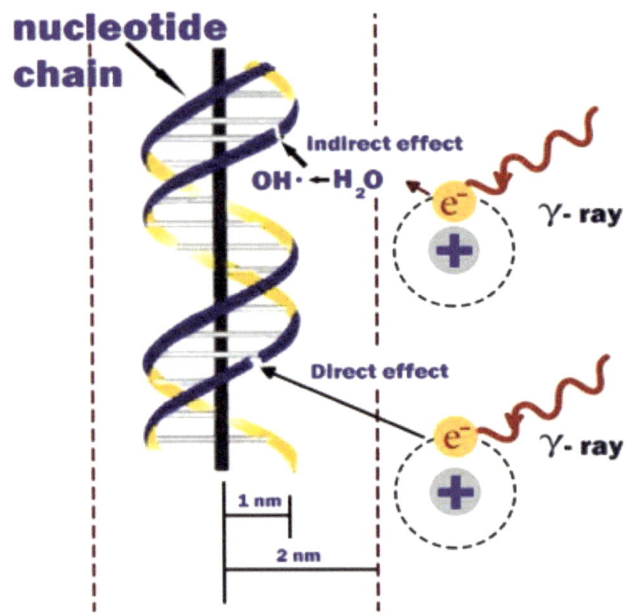

Figure 2.
Indirect versus direct DNA insults. Here is shown the direct effect of high-energy photons on the DNA backbone and the production of hydroxide free radicals that can then go on to react with the nucleic acids. Adapted from Desouky et al. [1].

2.2 Fractionation

Radiation doses delivered in external beam radiation therapy (EBRT) are measured in units called Gray (Gy), representing the absorption of 1 Joule per kilogram of tissue. In RT, doses may range from as small as 8 Gy for palliative purposes to as large as 81 Gy for definitive therapy in cases of prostate cancers. Administering higher doses of radiation in a single exposure poses significant risk to the normal tissues surrounding the tumor, potentially causing extensive damage to these cells in addition to targeted tumor cell death. To mitigate such risks, fractionation, or the division of the total radiation dose into smaller, individual doses, is commonly employed. Each fraction represents a single exposure, with the dose per fraction determined by dividing the total dose to be delivered by the number of fractions.

Fractionation offers several key advantages. By allowing intervals between treatments, normal tissues can repair themselves, which reduces the side effects associated with a radiation dose. Recall that normal cells possess mechanisms to repair DNA and cellular damage caused by radiation exposure, whereas many of these repair mechanisms are defective or absent in tumor cells [4]. Fractionation capitalizes on this biological disparity to deliver potent doses to tumors while minimizing severe side effects in normal tissue.

In planning radiation schedules, the biological effective dose (BED) is utilized to quantify the biological impact of a specific radiation treatment [5]. This metric considers not only the physical dose but also the fractionation schedule and the type of radiation employed, providing a comprehensive assessment of the treatment's biological efficacy. This concept helps provide a quantitative explanation for why the delivery of 30 Gy in 5 fractions can have a larger impact than the same dose divided over 10 or

15 fractions. A patient's radiation team utilizes various techniques to ensure the BED will be maximally efficacious as well as inflict minimal side effects for the patient.

2.3 Application to multidisciplinary cancer care

Patients diagnosed with most types of cancer should be promptly referred to Radiation Oncology upon diagnosis, as consideration for RT should be an integral component of the multidisciplinary care approach. Upon referral, patients will undergo evaluation by a specialized physician experienced in the use of RT for cancer treatment. RT offers a variety of uses and endpoints for patients, including curative intent, locoregional control, or palliation. RT has proved extremely efficacious in all of these endpoints and directly contributes to cure in 40% of cases who achieve this outcome [6].

RT with curative intent may serve as the primary local treatment, aiming to eliminate cancer cells without resorting to surgical intervention, or it may be combined with surgery. When RT is employed to avoid surgery altogether, it is termed definitive. Definitive RT is applicable to various cancers such as prostate cancer, head and neck cancers, lung cancer, or HCC. In conjunction with surgery, RT can be either performed adjuvantly (i.e., administered after surgery) or neoadjuvantly (i.e., given before surgery to facilitate easier tumor resection). For instance, breast cancer frequently requires adjuvant radiation with postoperative surgical bed or chest wall RT considered standard of care for optimal outcomes. Similarly, tumors of the gastrointestinal tract, such as colon or esophageal tumors, may benefit from neoadjuvant therapy, where RT aids in shrinking tumors to improve outcomes of curative resection.

RT is often combined with chemotherapy or immunotherapy to enhance the likelihood of cure. The combination of modalities can lead to mutual sensitization. For example, RT's killing of cancer cells can induce the release of tumor-associated antigens, which, when combined with tumor-directed immunotherapy, can augment the body's ability to mount an immune response [7]. The synergy that can be achieved by these modalities is often utilized in the treatment of lung cancer for example, which has led to great strides in survival in lung malignancies [8]. Similarly, chemotherapies arrest a cancer cell's capability to produce new nucleic acids or repair DNA damage, leading to sensitization of the tumor cells to DNA damage from RT.

A critical aspect often overlooked by care teams is the role of RT in the care of patients with primarily palliative intent. RT therapy is highly effective in alleviating pain secondary to metastatic disease, notably in bone metastases. RT can reduce tumor-associated pain in 60–80% of treated patients, with a third reporting complete resolution of pain [9]. Other palliative applications may include reducing focal symptoms from mass effect of intracranial tumors, reducing ulceration or from tumors invading the skin or GI tract, and even reducing airway compression or hemoptysis in lung malignancy [10].

Integrating RT into the treatment plan at the outset enhances cancer treatment strategies and overall outcomes for patients. This holds true in the case of HCC, as will be further discussed in subsequent sections of this chapter.

3. Stereotactic body radiation therapy in the treatment of hepatocellular carcinoma

While tumor resection and transplantation have been the mainstays of curative therapy for HCC for decades, only a minority of patients (approximately 30%)

are eligible for these treatments due to factors such as cancer stage, tumor size, or baseline liver function [11]. Other local therapies, such as radiofrequency ablation and trans-arterial chemoembolization (TACE), can also be utilized in select patients, offering significant survival benefits [12]. RT was not historically as widely used as other modalities until the early 2000s in the treatment of HCC. Before the advent of modern conformal RT technologies, whole and partial EBRT for liver cancer was associated with high rates of radiation-induced liver disease (RILD) [13]. The risk of classical presentations of RILD appeared to be minimal when radiation doses were kept below certain thresholds, but such constraints made achieving tumoricidal doses challenging [13].

However, in the 1990s, the development of multi-leaf collimators combined with CT-based treatment planning enabled RT to become much more targeted, sparing surrounding tissues from a majority of the delivered dose [13]. With the development of three-dimensional conformal RT (3D RT), more targeted radiation planning could offer higher doses to the tumor while simultaneously sparing surrounding tissues from RILD-inducing exposure. Tumor immobilization techniques also advanced the field as now there was a method of controlling for the organ motion associated with breathing [13]. The University of Michigan group showed that with 3D RT conventional fractionation, they were able to reach doses from 60 to 90 Gy while respecting acceptable dose constraints to normal tissues in patients with unresectable intrahepatic tumors [14, 15].

With even further advancement, SBRT emerged, allowing for large tumoricidal doses to be delivered in fewer fractions and with lower incidences of toxicities [13]. The development of SBRT marked a significant step forward in the technique of RT delivery. This step only became possible in the past 10–20 years alongside improvements in target visualization of the time of treatment (i.e., image-guided RT), ability to shape and conform RT doses tightly around target volumes, and computing capabilities that allowed such treatments to be planned efficiently. SBRT has since become a significant component of the standard treatment for numerous cancers including HCC. This section will discuss the technique of SBRT, the supportive literature, indications for clinical use, and the expected toxicities in patients undergoing liver SBRT.

3.1 Understanding stereotactic body radiation therapy

SBRT is a widely utilized method for delivering EBRT, usually utilizing photon-based external beam radiation. SBRT employs highly conformal treatment plans to administer significantly larger radiation doses per fraction (~6–10 Gy) as compared to conventional RT (1.8–2.2 Gy per fraction) [13]. This method can deliver higher doses compared to conventional EBRT and often can do so in 3–5 fractions instead of the typical 10–20 fractions. Utilizing advanced imaging techniques like CT scans, SBRT precisely targets the tumor, directing radiation beams from multiple angles along multiple planes to maximize tumor dose while minimizing exposure to healthy tissues [13].

SBRT finds particular utility in treating small to medium-sized tumors such as prostate adenocarcinoma, lung malignancies, and spinal tumors. It can be employed for definitive treatment of primary tumors or in managing limited metastatic disease, including spinal or lymph node disease. Early studies exploring SBRT included sites like the liver, lungs, and retroperitoneal space were first published in the late 1990s [16, 17]. The technology behind SBRT shares similarities with Stereotactic Radiosurgery (SRS), which is used for the treatment of intracranial disease. Today, both SBRT and SRS are daily tools in Radiation Oncology, treating a variety of common malignancies.

When planning SBRT, radiation oncologists work in a series of treatment volumes that represent tissues that are either to be targeted by the beams or to be avoided. Gross tumor volume (GTV) represents the actual tumor's volume as seen on imaging [18]. Typically, a margin around the GTV, called the planning target volume (PTV), is also delineated to ensure full dose coverage of the tumor while accounting for any errors in daily setup or tumor motion [18]. The goal of EBRT planning is to ensure the entire GTV and PTV receive at least 95% of the prescribed radiation dose while minimizing the dose to the tissues outside of these volumes. This can be accomplished by changing the angle of beams and the energy that each beam emits. **Figure 3** illustrates these planning components and their delineation in planning software. While the literature includes many treatment prescriptions and fractionation schemes, typically, SBRT plans include doses of 30–50 Gy in 3–5 fractions [19].

Often, fiducial markers can be placed in the tumor by a radiologist in order to help with targeting the GTV. Fiducial markers are small (3 mm) metal markers that are placed in or around the tumor by needles through image guidance. These are radiopaque and appear clearly on imaging and can be used to assist in target volume delineation and in ensuring accuracy during treatment delivery. More specifically, fiducials may be used either during initial set up of patient's during SBRT delivery, matching the position and orientation to that of initial CT simulation, or continuously through treatment for "real time" tumor tracking and accuracy during beam delivery.

Other volumes also include delineating the organs at risk (OARs). These are volumes that we hope to protect from radiation dose. For the liver, these may include healthy liver volume, the spinal cord, the kidneys, the stomach, and the ribs, among others. After these volumes are delineated by the physician and beam position and energies are planned, computer software can calculate the doses delivered to each

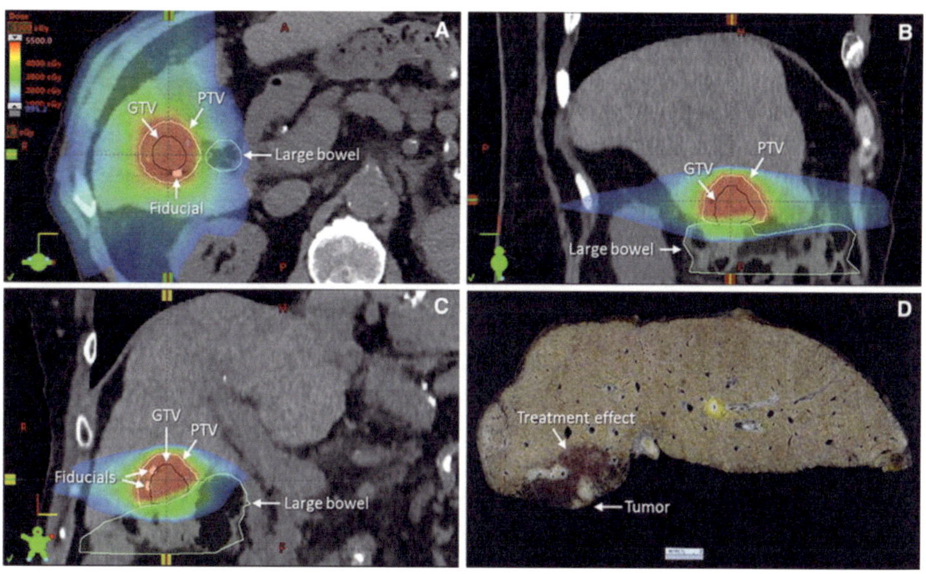

Figure 3.
(A, B, and C) here is shown an example of the outcome of planning SBRT for a 2 cm tumor identified on pathology as HCC. The prescribed dose was 50 Gy in 5 fractions. GTV and PTV volumes are delineated and labeled here. Surrounding the volumes are shades correlating to dose that they will be receiving. Tissues in red are receiving 100% of the dose; regions in green are receiving 50% (25Gy) of the dose, and those in blue are receiving 20% (10Gy) of the dose. (D) Shows a liver on cross section on autopsy after liver SBRT showing the necrosis and fibrosis of tissue included in the GTV and PTV. Adapted from Haddad et al. [18].

volume, including the OARs. Based on these calculations, the physician decides whether these doses are safe and efficacious enough to move forward with treatment or if the plan should be re-optimized to produce a better therapeutic ratio. Radiation oncologists use published tissue constraints for OARs that are often referred to for such clinical decisions. These list the doses that are maximally allowed for a healthy OAR to receive before the risk of toxicity becomes significant.

3.2 Indications and guidelines

Key to understanding the role of RT in HCC is identifying which patients are suitable for liver SBRT. Resection and transplantation remain the first-line therapies for early-stage HCC with normal liver function and in patients who are good candidates for surgery [20]. Surgery could involve resection of only affected lobes or liver transplant after total hepatectomy. Tumors smaller than 2 cm and patients without signs of portal hypertension are the most ideal candidates for resection followed by transplantation [20]. However, there is no upper limit of tumor size for surgical resection alone without transplantation, and it has been shown to confer a survival benefit. Thus, referral to a surgical oncologist should be considered for any patient presenting with HCC [21]. If the patient is not a candidate for surgery, other locoregional therapies should be considered, as HCC tends to remain confined to the liver. These can include ablation, arterially directed embolization, or radiotherapy.

Radiofrequency ablation (RFA) is a well-supported method of locoregional therapy but is most effective in tumors ≤3 cm and is often avoided if the tumor is near a major blood vessel [22]. Arterially directed embolization is also a well-supported localized treatment for HCC, working by blocking arterial blood flow to the tumor and inducing ischemia. Because HCC tumors primarily derive blood flow from the hepatic artery, whereas healthy liver parenchyma derive most of its perfusion from the portal circulation, this is an efficient and targeted way to starve tumor cells while sparing normal tissue [21]. TACE has no constraints in terms of tumor size but is generally avoided if the patient presents with portal venous thrombosis, as embolization of both components of the liver's dual blood supply would cause ischemia to normal tissues as well [21].

SBRT is a viable option for uni- or multifocal intermediate-stage hepatocellular carcinomas with or without vascular involvement [20]. Unlike RFA, SBRT does not have tumor size constraints and thus can be used in patients with larger tumors as long as dose constraints for the normal liver can be met and there is sufficient healthy liver for normal function [20]. A relative contraindication to SBRT would include Child-Pugh Class (CPC) -C liver function, as studies have shown CPC-C patients are at highest risk for RILD due to radiosensitivity of the tissue [20].

In advanced disease with extrahepatic spread and end-stage liver function, the role of RT is limited to the palliative setting. For extrahepatic spread, treatment with systemic therapies such as sorafenib or more recently combined targeted and immunotherapy (e.g. bevacizumab/atezolizumab) is the standard of care [20, 23]. Multidisciplinary input and shared decision-making with the patient should be emphasized in advanced disease, as some patients with poor functional status may prefer supportive care over anti-tumor therapy.

3.3 A review of SBRT as definitive therapy in hepatocellular carcinoma

A series of prospective studies published in the last 20 years have supported the use of SBRT in the definitive treatment of early or intermediate stage HCC. SBRT has been found to achieve excellent locoregional control (LC), demonstrate comparable overall survival rates compared to other local treatment methods, and exhibit minimal toxicity. This section provides a review of these seminal studies and discusses their implications for the current treatment of HCC in the radiation oncology suite.

Kwon et al. published one of the earliest phase II clinical trials on the use of SBRT for HCC [24]. They reported on 42 patients with HCC who were ineligible for surgery or RFA. Patients had to have CPC-A or -B disease and no prior history of RT. Each patient was treated with 30–39 Gy in 3 fractions. One- and three-year survival rates were 92.9 and 58.6%, respectively. They reported one patient died of hepatic failure, which may have been related to their RT, but no other significant toxicities were reported [24].

Kang et al. focused on 47 patients with inoperable HCC, including those with CPC-A or -B disease who had failed previous TACE treatment [25]. The inclusion criteria also limited tumor size to less than 10 cm and included patients with portal vein tumor thrombosis. SBRT was delivered in doses ranging from 42 to 60 Gy in 3 fractions. The authors reported a 2-year local control rate of 94.6% and an overall survival of 68.7%. Rates of grade 3 gastrointestinal toxicities were limited to 6.4%, with grade 4 toxicities at 4.3%. This trial established that salvage SBRT in patients with failed TACE treatment was well tolerated and provided excellent local control and overall survival [25].

Bujold et al. reported outcomes of a sequential Phase I and II clinical trials for SBRT in 102 patients with locally advanced HCC and CPC-A disease [26]. There was tumor vascular thrombosis in 55% of these patients, making them ineligible for TACE. Half of these patients had undergone previous local treatment including surgical resection, RAF, or TACE, and half were receiving SBRT as their primary definitive treatment. They delivered SBRT in doses of 24–54 Gy in 6 fractions. The authors reported no cases of RILD but did report progression to liver failure in 5 patients and a duodenal bleed in 1 patient, which may have been secondary to duodenal RT exposure. LC at 1 year was 87%, and one-year survival rate was 55% with median survival of 17 months. Compared to systemic therapy, which is the only other treatment option available for patients with tumor vascular thrombosis, SBRT was highly favorable as median survival for those on sorafenib is 7.9 months [23]. This study established that SBRT is a favorable option for patients with underlying tumor vascular thrombosis without otherwise advanced disease.

Lasley et al. then published a similar phase I and II clinical trial of 59 patients with nonresectable HCC with CP-A or -B disease [27]. Most of these patients (85%) had no prior local therapy. 20% of these patients had portal tumor vascular thrombosis, and the maximum tumor size for enrollment was 6 cm. This study delivered SBRT doses ranging from 36 to 55 Gy in 3 or 5 fractions and on average gave higher doses to CPC-B patients. Local control rates at 6 months for CPC-A patients was 92% and for CPC-B patients was 93% [27]. Median overall survival for CPC-A patients was 44.8 months and for CPC-B patients was 17.0 months. Notably, 12 patients experienced radiation-related grade III or IV liver toxicities, and 14% of CPC-B patients experienced RILD.

Studies comparing definitive RFA and SBRT have not made clear which option is preferable. Wahl et al. published a study of 224 patients with inoperable HCC who underwent RFA or SBRT retrospectively [28]. SBRT doses ranged from 27 Gy to 60 G in 5 fractions. Local control with RFA at 1 year was 83.6% and was 97.4% for those in the SBRT group. At 2 years, local control rates were 80.2 and 83.8% for RFA and SBRT, respectively [28]. Overall survival at one and 2 years were comparable for both groups. However, another study of 3980 patients from the National Cancer Database found 5-year overall survival to be higher in the RFA group as compared to the SBRT group (30 vs. 19%) [29]. Given the retrospective nature of these comparisons, both are susceptible to bias and should be interpreted with caution.

Finally, the recent TRENDY trial has compared TACE and SBRT in a small sample of 30 patients [30]. The trial closed early due to slow accrual but did publish their findings with the caveat of a small n-value. The authors found local control rates were improved in the SBRT group and saw no differences in overall survival or quality of life. They recommended international multicenter cooperation in future work to compare these two treatment options [30].

The combination of locoregional therapies has also been an area of investigation. When used together, the synergy of two treatment modalities should result in more effective tumor killing. Meng et al. reported on 1476 patients across 17 studies combining TACE and SBRT, showing improved survival rates compared to TACE alone [31]. More recently, early data has found that sequential systemic therapy following SBRT was more beneficial than systemic therapy alone [32]. The recently reported results of RTOG 1112, a phase III randomized controlled trial of sorafenib alone versus sorafenib and SBRT, has found an overall survival benefit from the addition of SBRT. Among patients receiving SBRT followed by sorafenib, the median overall survival was 15.8 months, compared to 12.3 months with sorafenib alone [32]. While this benefit was low, it was among a heavily pretreated population with a large percentage of patients showing macrovascular tumor thrombosis. Additionally, they found no significant difference in treatment-related gastrointestinal side effects between the groups, and in fact, quality of life scores were 10% higher in the sequential treatment group at 6 months with the addition of SBRT. These studies suggest the potential for future work to expand the use of SBRT in combination with other systemic or local therapies.

The current NCCN guidelines recommend SBRT be utilized when RFA and TACE are contraindicated or have failed [20]. Many questions remain to be answered in terms of which order locoregional therapies should be considered, or for which patients each therapy is optimal for. One currently open trial at Stanford University hopes to compare in patients who have recurrent or persistent disease after initial TACE whether further subsequent attempts at TACE or SBRT is more efficacious. A similar trial published from Italy demonstrated improved LC and PFS among patients treated with SBRT after failed TACE; however, this trial suffered from low accrual and high crossover from the TACE to SBRT arm, which may have diluted the impact of treatment arms on more concrete endpoints including overall survival [33].

Clearly, however, for many patients who have larger tumors with vascular involvement or unfavorable tumor location for ablation, SBRT is an efficacious and well-tolerated treatment option that can prolong life and provide excellent local control.

3.4 Dose: volume effects and toxicities

While SBRT is an effective local therapy with outstanding local control rates, as with any cancer therapy, one must consider the potential side effects and toxicities compared to the tumoricidal effect. Doses in SBRT are primarily limited by the surrounding healthy liver and nearby luminal gastrointestinal organs, such as the duodenum and stomach. The presence of HCC alone as compared to liver metastases increases the radiosensitivity of the surrounding normal liver, so this is a critical consideration [34].

Significant efforts have focused on understanding the impact of radiation exposure on liver function. RILD is categorized into two main diagnostic groups: "classical" and "nonclassical" disease. Classical RILD is characterized by hepatomegaly (without jaundice), elevated liver enzymes (especially alkaline phosphatase), and ascites within 3 months of RT [35]. Nonclassical disease represents any liver disease seen within the 3 months following RT other than classical RILD. Either condition can also present with other signs of liver dysfunction including coagulopathy, low serum albumin, elevations in serum bilirubin, and even in severe cases hepatic encephalopathy [35]. Gastrointestinal (GI) complications could include nausea, fatigue, gastritis, duodenal or gastric ulcers, colitis, and diarrhea [36].

The risk for developing RILD is much higher in preexisting disease (CPC- B or -C patients) as low baseline liver reserve leaves little room for loss of functional liver [35]. Wei et al. reported that hepatic function loss after SBRT for HCC was related to the dose delivered and is in part mediated by liver inflammation [37]. Their study concluded that regional differences in liver function can be mapped, and adjustments in dose arrangement in SBRT planning can mitigate damage to liver regions that are already partially compromised.

Radiation dose limits have been established that consider the dose-volume effects of SBRT and the risk of developing worsening liver function after specific doses of radiation [36]. After analysis of a number of studies, Miften et al. reported constraints to the mean liver dose (MLD), where dose to the entire volume of the patient's liver minus the GTV is calculated [36]. Here, they recommend for primary HCC, the MLD be less than 13 Gy in 3 fractions or less than 18 Gy in 6 fractions as this was associated with a less than 20% probability of developing grade III liver enzyme toxicities [36]. Other constraints for liver SBRT are based on the volume of liver that receives below a particular dose (i.e., a reserved cold volume). Son et al. suggested ensuring >800 cm^3 of normal liver should receive <18 Gy in 3–5 fractions [38]. For luminal GI organs such as the stomach or bowel, dose constraints primarily relate to maximal point dose rather than mean or volumetric dose constrain. Based on the constraints of the RTOG 1112 trial, for such organs doses during SBRT should limit the volume of stomach, small bowel, and duodenum exposed to greater than 30 Gy to 0.5 cc of the organ volume [39].

4. Proton beam therapy for hepatocellular carcinoma

Proton-based RT is a well-established method for treating various malignancies. Proton therapy has been extensively studied and found to be just as or in some instances more efficacious than photon therapy. Protons are particularly useful in the pediatric population in the treatment of tumors of the brainstem, paranasal sinuses, spinal cord, or skull base [40]. Studies have also shown proton therapy to efficacious in treating tumors of the prostate, lung, and breast, but often, protons are not significantly more efficacious options than traditional photon therapy for these disease sites unless under specific clinical circumstances.

The advantages of proton therapy stem from a unique property of protons that lowers dose delivered to the surrounding tissues. Depending on the energy of the beam, protons penetrate tissues to a specific depth, where they deposit all their energy into target tissues and exhibit minimal exit dose [40]. This point where the proton deposits its energy is known as the Bragg peak [40]. This characteristic allows for the sparing of tissues beyond the target depth, which is an advantage not achievable with photons. This decreased backscatter allows for less normal tissue irradiation and therefore allows for the delivery of higher doses to the tumor while avoiding toxicities. **Figure 4** depicts the differences in RT dose distributions between conventional RT, proton therapy, and SBRT [41]. This difference may be especially advantageous in patients with underlying liver disease wherein sparing of functional liver is critical to reducing the risk for RILD.

Doses in particle therapy, specifically protons, are denoted in Gray Equivalents (GyE). This measure is used because the relative biological effectiveness of photons versus protons differs. Proton beams have a slightly higher relative biological effect compared to photons for the same physical energy deposition (the relative biological effectiveness of protons to photons is about 1.1), so to measure doses that would be biologically equivalent to photons, we use GyE [42].

However, proton therapy is significantly more expensive than photon-based RT, and as such, its availability is comparatively limited. As of 2024, there are 44 proton centers in the United States and 89 worldwide [43, 44]. Despite these limitations, several trials have investigated the impact of proton therapy in treating HCC.

4.1 Protons in definitive therapy for hepatocellular carcinoma

While photon trials have shown enormous promise in terms of local control and survival, proton trials have been just as encouraging, if not slightly better. Fukumitsu et al. reported on 51 patients with Child-Pugh Class A or B HCC who were treated with 66 GyE in 10 fractions [45]. The study demonstrated promising overall survival rates, with 49.2% at 3 years and 38.7% at 5 years. Additionally, they achieved excellent local control rates of 94.5% at 3 years and 87.8% at 5 years. Proton therapy was well tolerated, with only grade I or II toxicities reported.

Hong et al. reported a Phase II multi-institutional study of proton therapy in patients with multiple forms of liver tumors, half of whom had HCC [46]. This study included patients with CPC- A and -B disease, and 27% had multiple hepatic HCC tumors. The median dose delivered was 58 GyE in 15 fractions. The overall survival

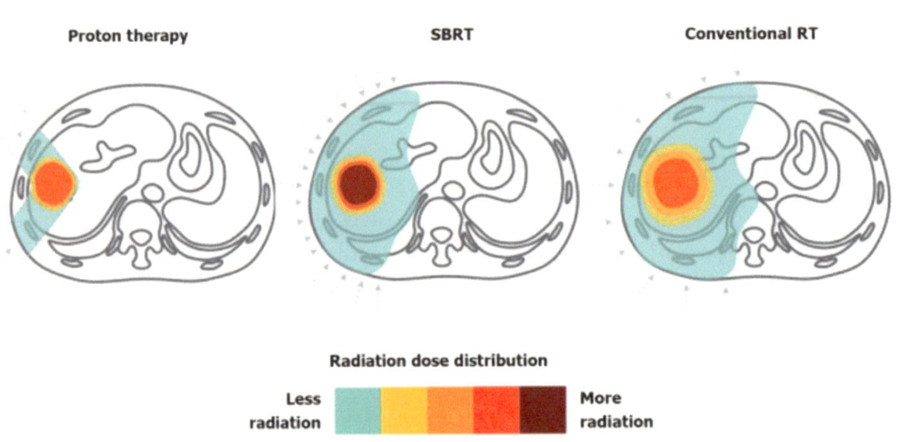

Figure 4.
Here, dose distributions are compared between the key methods of EBRT delivery discussed thus far. Proton therapy (left) has the least dose exposure in healthy surrounding tissue due to the Bragg peak properties of proton therapy. SBRT (middle) is also compared to conventional RT (right), which shows SBRT still has dose exposure to surrounding normal tissues, but less so than conventional EBRT. Adapted from Cheng et al. [41].

rate of HCC patients was 63.2% at 2 years, and the local control rate at the same time point was 94.8% [46]. They reported patients tolerated treatment well with few side effects.

Finally, a prospective multicenter study published by Mizumoto et al. followed 576 patients treated with protons across 12 centers in Japan [47]. They found the average overall survival time was 48.8 months and the median progression-free survival time was 14.7 months with 7.8% of patients developing local recurrence [47]. The complication rate at 27 months of follow-up was 4.7% the most common of which was liver failure in 7 patients.

While these studies paint a promising picture for proton therapy, as of yet, phase III randomized trials comparing proton beam therapy to photon therapy or other locoregional therapies have not been completed. However, for patients presenting to a center with proton capabilities, proton therapy is an efficacious option, particularly for those for whom RFA and TACE are not viable options.

5. Palliative radiotherapy

While much of this chapter has focused thus far on the ways in which RT is useful in the definitive treatment of HCC, it is important to discuss palliative RT, as 40% of referrals to the radiation oncology department are typically palliative in nature [48]. RT can have multiple roles in the care of patients whose prognosis does not include a possibility of cure. Often, RT offers a cost-effective, efficacious, and well-tolerated method of relieving pain or other consequences of local tumor growth. These could include pain, bleeding, weight loss, and the effects of local tumor mass effect. Common indications for palliative RT include painful metastatic disease to the bones, focal neurological symptoms secondary to tumor mass effect, and bleeding due to tumors in the lungs and stomach. In patients with end-stage HCC, palliative RT may be utilized to alleviate abdominal pain or discomfort, obstruction of the biliary tract, or in those who have painful bone metastases [49]. Here, we will discuss some of the data on these applications of palliative RT and discuss which patients are ideal for palliative RT.

5.1 Palliative RT in HCC related abdominal symptoms

Liver RT can be utilized in a palliative setting for patients with HCC experiencing abdominal or region-specific symptoms. Although not as extensively studied as other indications, it remains an important consideration for HCC patients. Trials investigating this indication have shown that even in advanced and incurable HCC, RT should be limited to patients with Child-Pugh Class A or B disease, as even lower palliative doses can lead to radiation-related toxicities in patients with Child-Pugh Class C disease [50]. Whole or partial liver RT has been well studied in patients with liver metastases secondary to colon cancer, as well as SBRT, which has been used to reduce tumor burden and alleviate pain. However, there is less research on these treatments for similar symptoms in the HCC population [50].

Several phase II trials have shown promising results in HCC patients receiving a single fraction of whole liver RT, with improvements in symptom management [51, 52]. A recent Phase III clinical trial by Dawson et al. has compared best supportive care alone to single fraction palliative RT (8 Gy) in 66 patients with HCC and liver metastases experiencing abdominal pain due to tumor burden [53]. The trial found that at 1 month follow-up, a significantly higher number of patients in the RT group reported "pain at its least" (63 vs. 28%) and reported pain relief on the Brief Pain Inventory (59 vs. 25%) [53]. Interestingly, the RT group also showed improved overall survival at 3 months compared to best supportive care (51 vs. 33%), indicating the potential benefit of single fraction palliative liver RT in advanced HCC patients with tumor-related abdominal pain and discomfort.

Palliative SBRT for painful HCC tumors has also shown promise quite recently. Sharma et al. reported in an observational retrospective study that 82.75% of 35 patients with advanced HCC, most of whom had portal IVC tumor thrombosis, experienced a reduction in pain, and 78% reported reductions in overall discomfort after SBRT [54]. Minimal toxicities and only slight worsening of liver function were observed. Future research comparing palliative SBRT to single fraction liver RT in HCC is warranted, but SBRT could be a valuable therapy for improving patient pain in advanced HCC in the future.

5.2 Palliative RT in bone metastases

Bone metastases are an extremely common indication for palliative RT. In patients with metastatic HCC, only 3–20% present with bone metastases, indicating that bone metastasis is rare compared to other tumors, such as breast, prostate, or lung tumors, which have very high rates of metastasis to the bone [55]. However, as HCC is relatively common, a large overall number of patients will still present with painful bone metastases secondary to cancer progression. As such, palliative RT for those with painful bone metastases is an important consideration in the multidisciplinary care of HCC patients.

Palliative therapy regimens for patients with painful bone metastases could include single fraction regimens of 8 Gy or multifractional regimens such as 30 Gy in 10 fractions. In either case, the response rates to pain from such palliative treatments are high. Hartsell et al. reported on a phase III trial of 898 patients with painful bone metastases randomized to either single fraction or multifractional palliative RT [56]. There was no statistical difference between these groups, but overall response to therapy was 66%. Of those who had a reduction in their pain level, about a third would report their pain totally resolved after either kind of RT [56].

Ultimately, in the treatment of bone mets, palliative RT is extremely well supported and has excellent response rates. Therefore, in advanced HCC patients presenting with painful bone mets, no matter their Child-Pugh Class, we recommend they be referred to the radiation oncology department for consideration for palliative radiation. This is a well-tolerated form of radiation that has few contraindications or toxicities. Thus, the radiation oncologist can serve a pivotal role in the palliative setting and improve the patients' quality of life tremendously.

6. Future directions

Finally, we will explore some innovative technologies that have recently emerged and may potentially revolutionize the treatment landscape for HCC in the coming decade. Specifically, we will delve into Adaptive RT and Biology-Guided RT, both of which represent recent significant advancements in treatment targeting. Despite the promising potential of these technologies, further research is needed to fully understand their impact on HCC treatment. Future studies should focus on elucidating the optimal patient selection criteria, treatment protocols, and long-term outcomes associated with Adaptive RT and Biology-Guided RT in HCC. If proven effective, these technologies could significantly enhance the therapeutic arsenal against HCC and improve the quality of life for patients facing this challenging disease.

6.1 Adaptive radiotherapy

Adaptive Radiotherapy first emerged as a possible avenue for improved RT planning in the late 1990s by Yan et al. who reported on its utility in the treatment of prostate cancer [57]. Adaptive RT is a cutting-edge technique that allows for real-time, day-to-day adjustments to radiation doses based on changes in the tumor's size, shape, and 3-D position. This approach ensures that the maximum dose is delivered to the tumor while minimizing damage to surrounding healthy tissue by accounting for daily anatomical differences.

CT or MRI images are taken while the patient is laying on the treatment table every day. This allows the radiation oncologist to redefine the location of the OARs and the tumor's location as these variables may vary somewhat on a day-to-day basis. The treatment software is then able to calculate the doses that each volume is going to receive and compare the adaptive treatment plan to the pre-planned treatment plan and allows the physician to choose the plan that maximizes tumor dose and minimizes OAR exposure.

Several studies have begun to investigate the efficacy of Adaptive RT in HCC treatment, with promising early results suggesting improved tumor control rates and reduced side effects compared to traditional RT approaches. The University of Michigan group reported a phase II study including 56 patients with HCC treated with adaptive SBRT [58]. Local control rates at 1 year follow-up were excellent with a recurrence rate of 6.4%. Using overlap weighting, they compared adaptive SBRT to conventional SBRT and found similar local control rates between the two methods; however, treatment-related toxicity risk was lower in the adaptive group with an impressive odds ratio of 0.26 [58]. Multiple pilot studies for using MRI-guided adaptive SBRT are collecting and preparing to publish their findings. As of yet, no phase III trials have compared adaptive SBRT to conventional SBRT.

6.2 Biology-guided radiotherapy

Biology-Guided RT involves the use of advanced imaging techniques and biomarkers to personalize radiation treatment based on the unique biological characteristics of the tumor. By targeting specific molecular pathways or genetic mutations driving tumor growth, Biology-Guided RT offers the potential for more effective and precise treatment strategies [59]. While still in the early stages of development, initial studies suggest that Biology-Guided RT may lead to improved outcomes and survival rates for HCC patients.

One example of biologically guided RT in HCC is the use of positron emission tomography (PET) imaging with tracers such as fluorodeoxyglucose to identify areas of high metabolic activity that correspond to the tumor [59]. This information can then be used to target these areas with higher doses of radiation while sparing surrounding healthy tissue. Work has been published examining the use of PET-guided therapy in prostate cancer, head and neck cancer, and lymphoma with promising results [60–62]. Future work will include examining the use of this methodology in SBRT planning for lung and gastrointestinal tumors. Some papers have examined using PET-guided therapy for directing the planning of simultaneous or integrated boosts during treatment for lung cancers and nasopharyngeal carcinomas [63, 64]. Using this method, boosts could be included in treatment planning to target lymph nodal metastasis in advanced HCC.

7. Conclusions

In the management of HCC, radiation therapy has emerged as a valuable noninvasive treatment option, particularly for early or intermediate tumors that are not amenable to resection, RFA, or TACE. SBRT can be utilized in patients with complications such as tumor vascular thrombosis or those with challenging anatomical locations. SBRT has proven to be safe and effective in these cases. Combining SBRT with arterially directed and systemic therapies has shown promise and may become a standard approach in the future, especially for patients with advanced disease. Proton therapy, though less accessible than photon-based SBRT due to limited availability of major proton centers, is an effective and safe alternative. Some work comparing SBRT to RFA has been done, but no clear evidence has proven one superior to the other. As such, both remain efficacious options for appropriate patients with intermediate or early HCC. However, RT may be considered relatively contraindicated in HCC patients with Child-Pugh Class-C disease due to the increased risk for RILD.

In cases of palliative disease, patients with painful metastases should be promptly referred for palliative radiation. This approach provides significant symptom relief in 60–70% of treated patients and improves the quality (and potentially quantity) of life. Palliative RT may also be useful in patients with abdominal pain secondary to HCC tumors, especially those with reasonable baseline liver function.

It is crucial for the patient's care team to include a radiation oncologist, as they play a pivotal role in the comprehensive treatment of HCC. It is important for clinicians treating HCC patients to be knowledgeable about the literature and indications for SBRT. These treatment options should be presented to eligible patients and discussed in multidisciplinary tumor boards to ensure comprehensive and effective care for all HCC patients.

Acknowledgements

We would like to acknowledge and thank St. Luke's University Health Network for their support of our work.

Conflict of interest

The authors declare no conflict of interest.

DOI: http://dx.doi.org/10.5772/intechopen.1005029

Author details

Christian N. Schill[1*] and William H. Smith[2]

1 Lewis Katz School of Medicine at Temple University, Bethlehem, PA, USA

2 Department of Radiation Oncology, St. Luke's University Health Network, Bethlehem, PA, USA

*Address all correspondence to: cnschill521@gmail.com

References

[1] Desouky O, Ding N, Zhou G. Targeted and non-targeted effects of ionizing radiation. Journal of Radiation Research and Applied Science. 2015;**8**(2):247-254

[2] Alizadeh E, Sanz AG, García G, Sanche L. Radiation damage to DNA: The indirect effect of low-energy electrons. Journal of Physical Chemistry Letters. 2013;**4**(5):820-825

[3] Jeggo PA, Löbrich M. DNA double-strand breaks: Their cellular and clinical impact? Oncogene. 2007;**26**:7717-7719

[4] Cornforth MN, Bedford JS. Ionizing Radiation Damage and its Early Development in Chromosomes. Cambridge, MA: Elsevier; 1993. pp. 423-496

[5] Dale RG, Jones B. The assessment of RBE effects using the concept of biologically effective dose. International Journal of Radiation Oncology, Biology, Physics. 1999;**43**(3):639-645

[6] Baskar R, Lee KA, Yeo R, Yeoh KW. Cancer and radiation therapy: Current advances and future directions. International Journal of Medical Sciences. 2012;**9**:193-199

[7] Gao Z, Zhao Q, Xu Y, Wang L. Improving the efficacy of combined radiotherapy and immunotherapy: Focusing on the effects of radiosensitivity. [Internet]. Radiation Oncology. 2023;**18**:89. Available from: https://ro-journal.biomedcentral.com/articles/10.1186/s13014-023-02278-5

[8] Zhang Z, Liu X, Chen D, Yu J. Radiotherapy combined with immunotherapy: The dawn of cancer treatment. Signal Transduction and Targeted Therapy. 2022;**7**:1-34

[9] Chow E, Harris K, Fan G, Tsao M, Sze WM. Palliative radiotherapy trials for bone metastases: A systematic review. Journal of Clinical Oncology. 2007;**25**:1423-1436

[10] Spencer K, Parrish R, Barton R, Henry A. Palliative radiotherapy. BMJ (Online). 2018;**360**:k821

[11] Delis SG, Dervenis C. Selection criteria for liver resection in patients with hepatocellular carcinoma and chronic liver disease. World Journal of Gastroenterology. 2008;**14**:3452-3460

[12] Hu Y, Zhao C, Ji R, Chen W, Shen Q, Chiang CL, et al. The role of stereotactic body radiotherapy in hepatocellular carcinoma: Guidelines and evidences. Journal of the National Cancer Center. Chinese National Cancer Center. 2022;**2**:171-182

[13] Dawson LA, Hashem S, Bujold A. Stereotactic body radiation therapy for hepatocellular carcinoma. American Society of Clinical Oncology Educational Book [Internet]. 2012;**32**:261-264. DOI: 10.14694/EdBook_AM.2012.32.171

[14] Dawson LA, McGinn CJ, Normolle D, Ten Haken RK, Walker S, Ensminger W, et al. Escalated focal liver radiation and concurrent hepatic artery fluorodeoxyuridine for unresectable intrahepatic malignancies. Journal of Clinical Oncology. 2000;**18**(11):2210-2218

[15] Ben-Josef E, Normolle D, Ensminger WD, Walker S, Tatro D, Ten Haken RK, et al. Phase II trial of high-dose conformal radiation therapy with concurrent hepatic artery floxuridine for unresectable intrahepatic malignancies. Journal of Clinical Oncology. 2005;**23**(34):8739-8747

[16] Blomgren H, Lax I, Näslund I, Svanström R. Stereotactic high dose fraction radiation therapy of extracranial tumors using an accelerator: Clinical experience of the first thirty-one patients. Acta Oncologica. 1995;**34**(6):861-870

[17] Blomgren H, Lax I, Göranson H, Kræpelien T, Nilsson B, Näslund I, et al. Radiosurgery for Tumors in the body: Clinical experience using a new method. Journal of Radiosurgery. 2004;**1**(1):63-74

[18] Haddad MM, Merrell KW, Hallemeier CL, Johnson GB, Mounajjed T, Olivier KR, et al. Stereotactic body radiation therapy of liver tumors: Post-treatment appearances and evaluation of treatment response: A pictorial review. Abdominal Radiology. 2016;**41**:2061-2077

[19] Ohri N, Tomé WA, Méndez Romero A, Miften M, Ten Haken RK, Dawson LA, et al. Local control after stereotactic body radiation therapy for liver Tumors. International Journal of Radiation Oncology, Biology, Physics. 2021;**110**(1):188-195

[20] NCCN Guidelines. NCCN clinical practice guidelines in oncology hepatocellular carcinoma. United States National Comprehensive Cancer Network. 2023. MS-20-31. Available from: https://www.nccn.org/guidelines/guidelines-detail?category=1&id=1514

[21] Crocetti L, Bargellini I, Cioni R. Loco-regional treatment of HCC: Current status. Clinical Radiology. 2017;**72**:626-635

[22] Weis S, Franke A, Berg T, Mössner J, Fleig WE, Schoppmeyer K. Percutaneous ethanol injection or percutaneous acetic acid injection for early hepatocellular carcinoma. Cochrane Database of Systematic Reviews. 2015;**2017**:CD006745

[23] Llovet JM, Ricci S, Mazzaferro V, Hilgard P, Gane E, Blanc JF, et al. Sorafenib in advanced hepatocellular carcinoma. New England Journal of Medicine. 2008;**359**(4):378-390

[24] Kwon JH, Bae SH, Kim JY, Choi BO, Jang HS, Jang JW, et al. Long-term effect of stereotactic body radiation therapy for primary hepatocellular carcinoma ineligible for local ablation therapy or surgical resection. Stereotactic radiotherapy for liver cancer. BMC Cancer. 2010;**10**:475

[25] Kang JK, Kim MS, Cho CK, Yang KM, Yoo HJ, Kim JH, et al. Stereotactic body radiation therapy for inoperable hepatocellular carcinoma as a local salvage treatment after incomplete transarterial chemoembolization. Cancer. 2012;**118**(21):5424-5431

[26] Bujold A, Massey CA, Kim JJ, Brierley J, Cho C, Wong RKS, et al. Sequential phase I and II trials of stereotactic body radiotherapy for locally advanced hepatocellular carcinoma. Journal of Clinical Oncology. 2013;**31**(13):1631-1639

[27] Lasley FD, Mannina EM, Johnson CS, Perkins SM, Althouse S, Maluccio M, et al. Treatment variables related to liver toxicity in patients with hepatocellular carcinoma, child-Pugh class a and B enrolled in a phase 1-2 trial of stereotactic body radiation therapy. Practical Radiation Oncology. 2015;**5**(5):e443-e449

[28] Wahl DR, Stenmark MH, Tao Y, Pollom EL, Caoili EM, Lawrence TS, et al. Outcomes after stereotactic body radiotherapy or radiofrequency ablation for hepatocellular carcinoma. Journal of Clinical Oncology. 2016;**34**(5):452-459

[29] Rajyaguru DJ, Borgert AJ, Smith AL, Thomes RM, Conway PD,

Halfdanarson TR, et al. Radiofrequency ablation versus stereotactic body radiotherapy for localized hepatocellular carcinoma in nonsurgically managed patients: Analysis of the national cancer database. Journal of Clinical Oncology. 2018;**36**(6):600-608

[30] Méndez Romero A, van der Holt B, Willemssen FEJA, de Man RA, Heijmen BJM, Habraken S, et al. Transarterial chemoembolization with drug-eluting beads versus stereotactic body radiation therapy for hepatocellular carcinoma: Outcomes from a Multicenter, randomized, phase 2 trial (the TRENDY trial). International Journal of Radiation Oncology, Biology, Physics. 2023;**117**(1):45-52

[31] Bin MM, Cui YL, Lu Y, She B, Chen Y, Guan YS, et al. Transcatheter arterial chemoembolization in combination with radiotherapy for unresectable hepatocellular carcinoma: A systematic review and meta-analysis. Radiotherapy and Oncology. 2009;**92**(2):184-194

[32] Dawson LA, Winter KA, Knox JJ, Zhu AX, Krishnan S, Guha C, et al. NRG/RTOG 1112: Randomized phase III study of sorafenib vs. stereotactic body radiation therapy (SBRT) followed by sorafenib in hepatocellular carcinoma (HCC). Journal of Clinical Oncology. 2023;**41**(4 Suppl.):489-489

[33] Comito T, Loi M, Franzese C, Clerici E, Franceschini D, Badalamenti M, et al. Stereotactic radiotherapy after incomplete transarterial (chemo-) embolization (TAE\TACE) versus exclusive TAE or TACE for treatment of inoperable HCC: A phase III trial (NCT02323360). Current Oncology. 2022;**29**(11):8802-8813

[34] Xu ZY, Liang SX, Zhu J, Zhu XD, Zhao JD, Lu HJ, et al. Prediction of radiation-induced liver disease by Lyman normal-tissue complication probability model in three-dimensional conformal radiation therapy for primary liver carcinoma. International Journal of Radiation Oncology, Biology, Physics. 2006;**65**(1):189-195

[35] Pan CC, Kavanagh BD, Dawson LA, Li XA, Das SK, Miften M, et al. Radiation-associated liver injury. International Journal of Radiation Oncology, Biology, Physics. 2010;**76**(3 Suppl.):S94-100

[36] Miften M, Vinogradskiy Y, Moiseenko V, Grimm J, Yorke E, Jackson A, et al. Radiation dose-volume effects for liver SBRT. International Journal of Radiation Oncology, Biology, Physics. 2021;**110**(1):196-205

[37] Wei L, Simeth J, Aryal MP, Matuszak M, Haken RKT, Cuneo K, et al. The effect of stereotactic body radiation therapy for hepatocellular cancer on regional hepatic liver function. International Journal of Radiation Oncology, Biology, Physics. 2023;**115**(3):794-802

[38] Son SH, Choi BO, Ryu MR, Kang YN, Jang JS, Bae SH, et al. Stereotactic body radiotherapy for patients with unresectable primary hepatocellular carcinoma: Dose-volumetric parameters predicting the hepatic complication. International Journal of Radiation Oncology, Biology, Physics. 2010;**78**(4):1073-1080

[39] Dawson LA, Winter K, Knox J, Zhu AX, Krishnan S, Guha C, et al. NRG/RTOG 1112: Randomized phase III study of Sorafenib vs. stereotactic body radiation therapy (SBRT) followed by Sorafenib in hepatocellular carcinoma (HCC) (NCT01730937). International Journal of Radiation Oncology*Biology*Physics. 2022;**114**(5):1057

[40] Paganetti H, Bortfeld T. Proton therapy. In: New Technologies in Radiation Oncology [Internet]. Berlin/Heidelberg: Springer-Verlag; 2006. pp. 345-363. Available from: http://link.springer.com/10.1007/3-540-29999-8_27 [Accessed: Feb 14, 2024]

[41] Chen LC, Lin HY, Hung SK, Chiou WY, Lee MS. Role of modern radiotherapy in managing patients with hepatocellular carcinoma. World Journal of Gastroenterology. 2021;**27**:2434-2457

[42] Paganetti H. Interpretation of proton relative biological effectiveness using lesion induction, lesion repair, and cellular dose distribution. Medical Physics. 2005;**32**(8):2548-2556

[43] National Association for Proton Therapy. Life saving. Life changing [Internet]. Available from: https://proton-therapy.org/ [Accessed: Mar 1, 2024]

[44] PTCOG. Facilities in operation [Internet]. Available from: https://www.ptcog.site/index.php/facilities-in-operation-public [Accessed: Mar 1, 2024]

[45] Fukumitsu N, Sugahara S, Nakayama H, Fukuda K, Mizumoto M, Abei M, et al. A prospective study of Hypofractionated proton beam therapy for patients with hepatocellular carcinoma. International Journal of Radiation Oncology, Biology, Physics. 2009;**74**(3):831-836

[46] Hong TS, Wo JY, Yeap BY, Ben-Josef E, McDonnell EI, Blaszkowsky LS, et al. Multi-institutional phase II study of high-dose hypofractionated proton beam therapy in patients with localized, unresectable hepatocellular carcinoma and intrahepatic cholangiocarcinoma. Journal of Clinical Oncology. 2016;**34**(5):460-468

[47] Mizumoto M, Ogino H, Okumura T, Terashima K, Murakami M, Ogino T, et al. Proton beam therapy for hepatocellular carcinoma: Multicenter prospective registry study in Japan. International Journal of Radiation Oncology, Biology, Physics. 2023;**118**(3):725-733

[48] Stavas MJ, Pagan JD, Varma S, Li B, Kachnic LA. Building a palliative radiation oncology program: From bedside to B.E.D. Practical Radiation Oncology. 2017;**7**(3):203-208

[49] Lutz ST, Jones J, Chow E. Role of radiation therapy in palliative care of the patient with cancer. Journal of Clinical Oncology: Official Journal of the American Society of Clinical Oncology. 2014;**32**:2913-2919

[50] Pennock M, Klein J, Lock M. Palliative radiotherapy for hepatic tumors: A narrative review of indications and recommendations. Annals of Palliative Medicine. 2023;**12**(6):1420-1446

[51] Yeung CSY, Chiang CL, Wong NSM, Ha SK, Tsang KS, Ho CHM, et al. Palliative liver radiotherapy (RT) for symptomatic hepatocellular carcinoma (HCC). Scientific Reports. 2020;**10**(1):1254

[52] Soliman H, Ringash J, Jiang H, Singh K, Kim J, Dinniwell R, et al. Phase II trial of palliative radiotherapy for hepatocellular carcinoma and liver metastases. Journal of Clinical Oncology. 2013;**31**(31):3980-3986

[53] Dawson LA, Fairchild AM, Dennis K, Mahmud A, Stuckless TL, Vincent F, et al. Canadian cancer trials group HE.1: A phase III study of palliative radiotherapy for symptomatic hepatocellular carcinoma and liver metastases. Journal of Clinical Oncology. 2023;**41**(4_Suppl.):LBA492-LBA492

[54] Sharma D, Thaper D, Kamal R, Yadav HP. Role of palliative SBRT in Barcelona clinic liver cancer-stage C hepatocellular carcinoma patients. Strahlentherapie und Onkologie [Internet]. 2023;**199**(9):838-846. Available from: https://link.springer.com/10.1007/s00066-023-02065-x

[55] Kim S, Chun M, Wang H, Cho S, Oh YT, Kang SH, et al. Bone metastasis from primary hepatocellular carcinoma: Characteristics of soft tissue formation. Cancer Research and Treatment. 2007;**39**(3):104

[56] Harstell WF, Scott CB, Bruner DW, Scarantino CW, Ivker RA, Roach M, et al. Randomized trial of short- versus long-course radiotherapy for palliation of painful bone metastases. Journal of the National Cancer Institute. 2005;**97**(11):798-804

[57] Yan D, Vicini F, Wong J, Martinez A. Adaptive radiation therapy. Physics in Medicine and Biology. 1997;**42**(1):123-132

[58] Herr DJ, Wang C, Mendiratta-Lala M, Matuszak M, Mayo CS, Cao Y, et al. A phase II study of optimized individualized adaptive radiotherapy for hepatocellular carcinoma. Clinical Cancer Research. 2023;**29**(19):3852-3858

[59] Shirvani SM, Huntzinger CJ, Melcher T, Olcott PD, Voronenko Y, Bartlett-Roberto J, et al. Biology-guided radiotherapy: Redefining the role of radiotherapy in metastatic cancer. British Journal of Radiology. 2021;**94**:20200873

[60] Freeman CL, Savage KJ, Villa DR, Scott DW, Srour L, Gerrie AS, et al. Long-term results of PET-guided radiation in patients with advanced-stage diffuse large B-cell lymphoma treated with R-CHOP. Blood. 2021;**137**(7):929-938

[61] Gaudreault M, Chang D, Hardcastle N, Jackson P, Kron T, Hofman MS, et al. Evaluation of PSMA-PET biology-guided radiotherapy sequential boost to the PSMA-avid subvolume in the prostate region in low-volume advanced prostate cancer. International Journal of Radiation Oncology*Biology*Physics. 2021;**111**(3):S52

[62] Gouw ZAR, La Fontaine MD, Vogel WV, van de Kamer JB, Sonke JJ, Al-Mamgani A. Single-Center prospective trial investigating the feasibility of serial FDG-PET guided adaptive radiation therapy for head and neck cancer. International Journal of Radiation Oncology, Biology, Physics. 2020;**108**(4):960-968

[63] Li QS, Liang N, Ouyang WW, Su SF, Ma Z, Geng YC, et al. Simultaneous integrated boost of intensity-modulated radiation therapy to stage II-III non-small cell lung cancer with metastatic lymph nodes. Cancer Medicine. 2020;**9**(22):8364-8372

[64] Qiu J, Lv B, Fu M, Wang X, Zheng X, Zhuo W. 18F-Fluoromisonidazole positron emission tomography/CT-guided volumetric-modulated arc therapy-based dose escalation for hypoxic subvolume in nasopharyngeal carcinomas: A feasibility study. Head & Neck. 2017;**39**(12):2519-2527